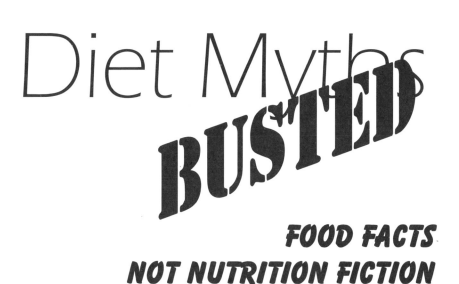

Diet Myths BUSTED

FOOD FACTS
NOT NUTRITION FICTION

Ann A. Rosenstein

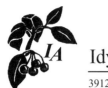

Idyll Arbor, Inc.

39129 264th Ave SE, Enumclaw, WA 98022 (360) 825-7797

Idyll Arbor Editor: Thomas M. Blaschko
Drawings: Ann A. Rosenstein
Back Cover Photo: Leo Rosenstein

ISBN: 9781882883837

Printed in the United States of America

Library of Congress Cataloging-in-Publication Data

Rosenstein, Ann A., 1958-
  Diet myths busted : food facts not nutrition fiction / Ann A. Rosenstein.
    p. cm.
  Includes bibliographical references and index.
  ISBN 978-1-882883-83-7 (alk. paper)
  1.   Nutrition--Popular works. 2.   Diet--Popular works. 3.   Health--Popular works. I. Title.
  RA784.R666 2011
  613.2--dc22
                                                      2010041437

*This book is dedicated to my many class participants
who have provided source material for this book,
all my clients that have shared their successes with me,
and to so many others who seek the truth about diet
and nutrition in the sea of hype and misinformation we
all live in.*

Contents

Acknowledgements

This book is based on the questions and concerns my clients, class participants, friends, and relatives have shared with me about nutrition and diet. In over 20 years of teaching, I have received hundreds of questions about what to do, what to eat, how to eat, how much, and when.

I want to thank my daughter Sarah who is a degreed, certified personal trainer, my son Ben who is graduating in Biomedical Engineering and stays fit on the Minnesota Crew team, and my husband Leo who also is a fitness instructor, for all of their input, suggestions, and hours of proofreading. I would also like to thank my editor and publisher Tom Blaschko for all his hard work, faith, and patience for taking a chance on what we hope is not just another diet book.

INTRODUCTION

A balanced diet is a cookie in each hand.
— Barbara Johnson

Keep everything as simple as possible but not simpler.
— Albert Einstein

As a certified fitness instructor and personal trainer for over 20 years, I am constantly asked questions by clients on how to lose weight, lose body fat, gain more muscle, what to eat, what not to eat, when to exercise, how to exercise, and the biggest question of all, how much is enough.

What is very clear is that most of us are bombarded with so much information and misinformation that we no longer know what to think. The result is that we become frustrated and discouraged as more and more "quick fixes" are introduced by the news media and bookstores, often contradicting what was said or introduced just a year or two ago.

Some may think that since I am not a doctor or a certified nutritionist, who am I to write about the myths of nutrition? I know what I see and what I have learned. My training and experience as a professional fitness instructor has given me valuable knowledge, experience, and insight.

Unlike other authors, I am not selling my brand of meal-replacement bars, exercise equipment, or recipes. I hope to dispel some of the most commonly held myths and ideas that seem to permeate all levels of the fitness and nutrition industry and to give you the tools and information you need to make eating and exercising an informed, rewarding, and beneficial experience.

Unlike other authors, I am not selling my brand of meal-replacement bars, exercise equipment, or recipes

Let me make one important thing clear right up front. All I am offering here is information. I am not suggesting a particular diet or a particular kind of exercise. If you are reading this and think you might want to make a change toward a healthier lifestyle, consult your health care professional. I can help you decide to make a change and I can give you information so you can make better decisions, but you are a unique person with your own personal situation. Consult an expert who knows YOU before making any radical changes, especially if there are concerns about your health.

□ ■ □ ■ □

Who needs this book? We all do! The doctors, nurses, and nutritionists in my classes are just as overweight and confused as the rest of the population. One of my clients, who struggles with her weight, went to a doctor who specializes in obesity. She walked in, noticed he was not only overweight but was obese, and promptly walked out. She asked me, "How can I take direction from him when he obviously needs some himself?"

Our daughter is studying to be a nurse. Her nutrition professor was a woman just over five feet tall who weighed almost 300 pounds. Again, our daughter wondered, "What is she doing teaching such a course? She certainly isn't a role model." Being a professional isn't a buffer against bad advice or poor habits.

Being a professional isn't a buffer against bad advice or poor habits.

□ ■ □ ■ □

Americans worry more than any other people on Earth about how our food and exercise habits will impact our health, yet we suffer more diet and sedentary-related health problems than people in most other countries. Being overweight or obese has become epidemic in America, affecting 66.7% of the population and it is getting worse. People who are obese now outnumber people who are overweight. Let me just put that in glaring numbers: as of July 2008 the population of the United States was 303,824,640 and the number of inactive people with poor diets was 215,160,000, leaving only 88,664,640 people who were active and healthy, less than 30% of the total. If nothing changes and the trend of the past three decades continues, by the year 2038, 86% of American adults will be overweight (51% of those obese).

Not only will waistlines expand, but health care costs will expand as well. At this moment, annual U.S. health care costs total $617 billion. By 2030, weight-related health care costs will total $957 billion, or $1 of every $6 spent on health care in the U.S. This means that the health care needs of an overweight or obese elderly person on Medicare will cost 17% more than the health care needs of an elderly person who is at a healthy weight.

For the first time since Man walked the Earth, the current obesity epidemic has produced a generation of people who are expected to have an overall life expectancy less than their parents. Until the

For the first time in world history, people who are malnourished and overweight outnumber people who are malnourished and underweight.

generation after the baby boomers, life expectancy increased steadily. For the first time in world history, people who are malnourished and overweight outnumber people who are malnourished and underweight.

Obesity and the Environment

The increase in obesity has been fueled by a complex interaction between behavioral, social, economic, and environmental factors that impact the population's genetic susceptibility. Food is abundant and

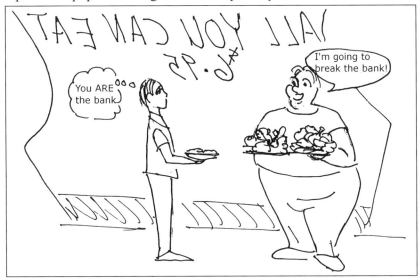

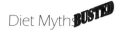

physical activity has become unnecessary. Our physiology requires physical movement as a means of maintaining equilibrium between energy in and energy out. Lack of exercise and too much available food are the basic problems. Genetic predisposition to being overweight is not enough of a factor to account for the sudden rapid rise of obesity.

There is just no way around it; if we want to maintain an effective, efficient body at an optimal weight, we have to engage in physical activity and fuel our bodies with whole-some nutrition in appropriate amounts. Does this mean we can't have pizza, hot dogs, ice cream, chocolate cake, beer, or a margarita? No! It means they become treats to be savored sparingly, not staples of the diet! Even an occasional fast-food meal is fine but becomes a problem, just like eating unhealthy food and/or overconsuming any food, when it is habitually chosen, rather than occasionally. How we choose what we eat is the question and the problem.

> *Does this mean we can't have pizza, hot dogs, ice cream, chocolate cake, beer, or a margarita? No!*

Brief History of Diets

Dieting has been around for thousands of years, but not in any struc-tured way like we see today. Dieting wasn't very common until the 1800s because overweight people were not common. Rich merchants, various ranks of royals, and other wealthy people were sometimes overweight. The rest of the population usually had to struggle to get enough food for their families' health; many were undernourished and physically exhausted. Being overweight was not a problem most people had, but many wished they did because it was an outward sign of success, pros-perity, and plenty.

Whenever a royal or other per-son of wealth decided that their inability to move around freely due to their weight was a problem, they reduced the quantity of their food consumption or hired people to do the work they couldn't. For example, when Henry VIII became too heavy

> *When Henry VIII became too heavy to mount his horse, rather than try to reduce his size, he had a crane made to hoist him up onto his horse*

to mount his horse, rather than try to reduce his size, he had a crane made to hoist him up onto his horse. In time, as living conditions improved, wealth was redistributed, allowing those lower down the economic scale more that was previously unavailable to them, such as excess food and drink. They also began to put on excess weight.

The human body is genetically predisposed to accumulate weight. Fatty and sugary foods are greedily digested by the body and the excess calories are stored by the body for a time when food may not be available. This survival system evolved over millions of years to offset the enormous number of people who must have starved to death due to a scarcity of food and nutrition.

Our bodies' survival mechanism against starvation is to store energy as fat. Biologically, modern men and women are no different from our prehistoric ancestors. A century or two of accessible food for all is not enough time to undo the eons of humans struggling to survive on barely enough. The human body has not had enough time to adjust to the modern realities of the abundance of food in developed countries. Since we know we are capable of storing more than we need, we must learn to consume food differently. Rising levels of cholesterol, blood pressure, cancers, heart disease, and other chronic diseases and conditions associated with obesity have become major problems, killing us off with increasing frequency. Yet people are still eating more, weighing more, dieting more, and getting more confused and frustrated.

> *The human body has not had enough time to adjust to the modern realities of the abundance of food in developed countries.*

To help illustrate the confusion let's look at a timeline of the more common dieting methods in recent history:

1930s —

- The Hollywood Diet, soon to be known as the Grapefruit Diet, was introduced.
- Seaweeds, such as kelp and bladderwrack, were promoted as foods of choice to end weight problems.

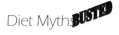

- "Diet guru" Victor Lindlahr regularly broadcast on national radio to spread news of "reverse calorie foods." He claimed he had discovered a catabolic system of weight loss where some foods supposedly used up more calories in being digested than they gave to the body.

1940s and 1950s —

- "Ideal weight" charts were created by matching weight with sex, height, and frame size.
- Amphetamine-derived diet pills were introduced and were soon found to be dangerous.

1960s —

- Jean Nidetch and her friends held a meeting in her apartment to share support and advice on dieting, thus beginning Weight Watchers.
- Dr. Atkins released his plan for weight loss. The high-protein, high-fat, and low-carbohydrate diet caused a storm of controversy that still rages today as multiple health fears and myths are voiced by critics.

1970s —

- The Food and Drug Administration (FDA) called for a ban on saccharin, an artificial sweetener, in the United States. Because of voter fury, the U.S. Congress did not heed this advice.
- The Pritikin Diet Program, endorsing low fat and high fiber, was introduced for those with heart conditions, but quickly was taken up by others for weight loss.
- The eating disorder, anorexia nervosa, was recognized for the first time as a health problem, as many continual dieters were becoming underweight.
- A new diet drug, fenfluramine, which makes the brain think the stomach is full, was introduced.

- Dr. Robert Linn invented a protein drink called Prolinn from slaughterhouse byproducts such as crushed horns, hooves, and hides that are treated with artificial flavorings and enzymes. In *The Last Chance Diet* he urged all those looking to lose weight to completely omit food and break their fast only by the use of his product. Somewhere around three million people gave it a go.
- In their book, *Fit for Life*, Harvey and Marilyn Diamond claimed that the human body's physiological needs for certain foods changes depending on the time of day.

1980s —

- The Beverly Hills Diet became the latest dieting craze, holding that only fruit should be eaten for the first ten days of the plan.
- An anti-diabetes system called the Glycemic Index was developed by Dr. David Jenkins and a team of scientists at the University of Toronto. To help simplify the problems suffered by diabetics, this index charts how quickly a range of diverse foods affects blood sugar levels. It was embraced by most diabetes organizations around the world, to help them better understand the impact of sugary and starchy carbohydrates. This system was soon misused by authors of fad diets to back up their weight loss claims.
- The TV personality, Oprah Winfrey, lost almost 70 pounds on a liquid diet.
- The health writer, Susan Powter, advised her female readers to diet less and exercise more.

1990s —

- The FDA demanded that food labeling should include more detailed information about calorie and fat content to assist dieting consumers and for better public health.
- A shocking report indicated that 40% of American children aged 9-10 years were dieting to lose weight.

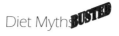

- Diet pills containing fenfluramine and dexfenfluramine were withdrawn by their manufacturers after the FDA reports that they cause valvular heart disease.

2000s —

- Some researchers claimed that, for the first time in recorded human history, the number of underfed people in the world has been exceeded by those that are overweight.

And so it goes. As the wealth of the world increases, our weight will also continue to increase unless we take measures to change it.

What to take away

- For the first time in history, our current lifestyle is reversing our longevity gains.
- The information out there is conflicting and confusing.
- We have the power and ability to reverse our current situation.

1. THE GENDER MYTH

Never trust a fat dietitian.

— Anonymous

MYTH: More women are overweight or obese than men.

WHY WE THINK THAT: Since most of the U.S. population is above normal weight and we see more women than men out and about, we assume women are more overweight or obese.

THE FACTS: Just look at the chart below: more men are overweight or obese than women. This is because women tend to care more about how they look than men. All you have to do is look at any mall directory. The stores devoted to women and their appearance; jewelry stores, shoe stores, clothing stores, stores that sell perfumes, and stores that sell lingerie, substantially outnumber the stores devoted to men. Throughout the country there are 9500 women-only health clubs. General health clubs have more female members than male, and women comprise well over half the participants in group fitness classes.

Even so, whether or not more men are overweight or obese than women, it is clear that the majority of our entire population is over-

It is clear that the majority of our population is overweight or obese.

weight or obese. An unhealthy population is unproductive and creates costly health care issues.

Table 1: 2005 Overweight and Obesity Rates for Adults by Gender[1]

State	Male (%)	Female (%)
Alabama	71.2	54.3
Alaska	69.6	54.8
Arizona	62.3	44.8
Arkansas	70.2	54.2
California	65.9	50.1
Colorado	61.5	43.0
Connecticut	67.6	43.9

State	Male (%)	Female (%)
Delaware	69.6	52.1
District of Columbia	56.8	48.1
Florida	69.0	48.1
Georgia	67.3	53.9
Hawaii	62.2	40.8
Idaho	68.7	48.1
Illinois	65.9	50.9
Indiana	68.4	51.2
Iowa	70.0	50.9
Kansas	67.0	49.4
Kentucky	70.3	55.1
Louisiana	69.9	55.2
Maine	65.3	49.1
Maryland	67.1	50.2
Massachusetts	64.4	42.5
Michigan	68.6	52.9
Minnesota	69.4	49.9
Mississippi	70.8	59.6
Missouri	70.9	59.6
Montana	65.5	44.2
Nebraska	69.8	51.1
Nevada	68.5	43.6
New Hampshire	68.9	46.5
New Jersey	64.3	47.0
New Mexico	65.5	51.3
New York	64.4	50.0
North Carolina	66.1	53.0
North Dakota	72.6	51.6
Ohio	69.5	51.8
Oklahoma	68.9	52.8
Oregon	64.7	48.5
Pennsylvania	69.1	50.2
Rhode Island	65.5	47.1
South Carolina	70.9	54.4

State	Male (%)	Female (%)
South Dakota	71.3	50.4
Tennessee	68.0	51.3
Texas	68.3	49.6
Utah	63.2	45.6
Vermont	63.9	45.1
Virginia	69.2	49.2
Washington	65.6	47.7
West Virginia	71.1	56.7
Wisconsin	69.3	49.3
Wyoming	69.6	49.6
United States	67.3	50.2

What to take away

- More men are overweight or obese than women.
- The problem of weight gain is getting worse.
- The majority of the U.S. population is overweight.

2. DIETING

Thank you for calling the Weight Loss Hotline. If you'd like to lose a half pound right now, press 1 eighteen thousand times.
— Randy Glasbergen

Each year millions of people go on diets, including fad diets, hoping to lose pounds and gain a slimmer, trimmer, healthier body. Ask anybody if they are dieting and, more often than not, they will say they are on a diet, need to go on a diet, or have just been on a diet. We try low-fat diets, protein diets, milkshake diets, low-carb diets, and even diets that limit us to one food group like the grapefruit diet or the cabbage diet. Many lose weight quickly and believe in the success of the diet. Unfortunately, most of us will not only regain the weight we lost but gain additional pounds as well. The premise of any diet is to eat less than we previously ate before going on a diet.

In reality, we are all on some kind of diet. If a person eats 4,000 calories a day of junk, that is their diet. If a person eats a reasonable

In reality, we are all on some kind of diet.

amount of food, such as 2,000 calories from wholesome sources, that is their diet. "Diet" refers to whatever we consistently eat. It doesn't matter which "diet plan" we choose to follow because as long as we consume less than we use we will lose weight. Once we have reached our desired weight, if we then resume our previous level of consumption, we will regain all that we lost. In today's language, dieting is a feast or famine method of eating that is a temporary way of consuming less food in the hopes of accomplishing a permanent goal. It's the temporary part that is a problem.

MYTH: Dieting works.

WHY WE THINK THAT: When we have a special event coming up, we pay attention to how we want to present ourselves and become more aware of what we eat and we see the results. We are also inundated with diet plans that promise, and even guarantee, weight loss.

THE FACTS: Diets, as a temporary way of eating, can work as a means of providing weight loss. They force us to pay attention to what we put into our mouths, how much we put into our mouths, when we put it in, and why. Diets also absolve us of our responsibility to think for ourselves. The diets, be they low-carb, low-fat, full of grapefruit, Weight Watchers, Jenny-Craig, or any other major diet program, all have it mapped out for us, so all we need to do is follow the instructions. However, many diets are so restrictive in their methods and in what types of foods they allow that it becomes increasingly boring and tedious to stick to them. Some are deficient in nutrition, so our bodies demand that we eat more. Since we have starved ourselves, we usually overeat and regain the weight we have lost. Many diet methods do try to educate us in the proper way to eat but, as many have witnessed, the information is confusing, ever changing, and often contradictory.

Here are eight basic reasons why "dieting" as the only way we try to lose weight doesn't work:

1. Fad diets are not permanent solutions to long-term weight problems. They are quick fixes that offer a false promise. We may lose weight

Fad diets are not permanent solutions to long-term weight problems.

initially, but as soon as we begin to eat regular food again or resume our previous eating habits, we regain the weight. The basic long-term problems are our eating habits and lack of activity. Until we begin exercising regularly and eating fewer calories and healthier foods, our weight will continue to go up and down. This is often referred to as yo-yo dieting.

2. Fad diets can upset our metabolism. Our metabolism is the rate at which our body burns calories. Our age and activity level determine how our body burns calories. In its normal state of homeostasis, the body learns to maintain the weight we normally carry. We all have a basal metabolic rate (BMR), the number of calories we burn at rest. Once we dramatically decrease calorie intake, our body will create a new BMR based on the lower calorie intake and lower body mass and our homeostasis will change. This means that when we resume eating the way we did at our previous level, we will gain back more weight than before because our body adjusted itself to surviving on fewer calories to fuel

less body mass. Losing weight slowly by following a healthy diet with foods in smaller amounts will keep our metabolism working properly.

3. Most fad diets concentrate on what foods we eat instead of what exercise we need. By just eliminating calories and not exercising, we may lose a few pounds but we are not replacing lost fat with lean muscle. Instead, we are losing both fat and lean muscle. Without lean muscle mass, our body looks flabby no matter how thin we are and we don't have the ability to burn calories efficiently. An exercise program along with a healthy diet will make us look leaner and trimmer and burn calories at an accelerated rate. Replacing lost fat with lean muscle allows our bodies to burn more calories at a faster rate, even at rest.

> *An exercise program along with a healthy diet will make us look leaner and trimmer.*

4. Some fad diets promote consuming little or no fat. Our body burns fat for energy. The philosophy behind these types of fad diets is, if we don't eat fat, then our body will burn its excess fat for energy, thus causing us to lose weight. Unfortunately, when we begin to starve our body of nutrients, it reverts to starvation mode and hangs onto stored fat. Then our body begins burning muscle for energy to compensate for the lack of nutrients. Once we go off the diet, our body will begin storing all excess calories as fat, making our body regain fatty tissue quicker. The loss of muscle reduces our ability to burn calories, making it easier to gain additional weight at a faster rate. Our body requires a variety of vitamins, minerals, proteins, carbohydrates, and fats to function properly and stay healthy. Remember, lean muscle burns calories and fat tissue stores calories. If we lose lean muscle mass, we lose our ability to burn calories; if we replace our lost muscle tissue with fat tissue, we improve our ability to store calories, meaning that we gain weight.

5. Many diets concentrate on the three-meal-a-day concept, leaving people hungry between meals. It usually isn't those three meals that sabotage a diet, it's the hunger in between. Snacking when very hungry leads to overeating and causes people to eventually give up the diet. People who eat several

> *It usually isn't those three meals that sabotage a diet, it's the hunger in between.*

small, healthy meals and snacks a day tend to maintain their weight better while keeping their energy levels up. Those who diet this way also have more success in losing weight because they are less tempted to cheat. This is because they never feel like they have to wait for the next time to eat, so they don't feel deprived of food.

6. Fad diets concentrate on losing weight too quickly. The initial weight we lose is water weight, fooling us into believing we are losing unwanted fat. When we resume eating what we think are regular amounts, the water weight comes back, too. To lose weight effectively, weight loss should be a gradual process.

7. Many fad diets limit carbohydrates. The body extracts energy from fat with the help of carbohydrates. Carbohydrates from natural sources, such as fruits and vegetables, help muscles use fat for

> *Our bodies are programmed to need a certain amount of protein and we will eat until that need is met.*

energy. Natural carbohydrates are actually good for us, even when we are trying to lose weight. Other diets limit protein. Our bodies are programmed to need a certain amount of protein and we will eat until that need is met. If protein sources are limited, we will meet our protein needs even if it means overeating or cannibalizing our own body's tissue.

8. Fad diets can be unhealthy for our body in the long run. By depriving our body of the nutrients it needs for long periods of time, we run the risk of damaging bones, vital organs, and even brain tissue. If we cycle, over and over, between losing and gaining significant amounts of weight, we will put stress on our immune system, heart, and lungs. We must lose weight slowly, using a healthy diet and an exercise program that become life-long habits as part of a healthy lifestyle. This really is the best and healthiest way to lose the pounds and stay fit for a lifetime.

MYTH: All I have to do is not give in to my cravings.

WHY WE THINK THAT: We believe that all we need to do is exercise willpower.

THE FACTS: There are three reasons this doesn't work. The first is that suppressing food cravings by exercising willpower can prove an overwhelming and self-defeating task. It is like trying to get the lyrics of

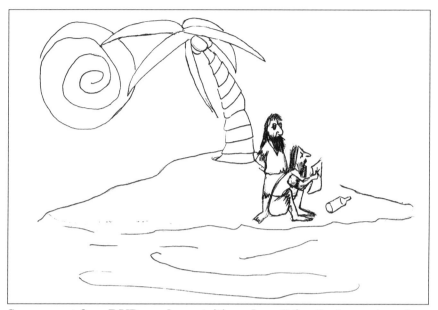

Says we get four DVDs and a nutrition plan all for the low price of $49 plus free shipping and handling.

a song out of our head. The more we try to suppress the lyrics, the more we end up having the tune run through our mind. Similarly, the longing for a cream-filled doughnut can nag at us for hours.

The second reason is that repeatedly succumbing to our every gastronomic desire negatively affects us. When we are pleasured with food, dopamine, a neurotransmitter, floods our body and makes us feel relaxed and satisfied. It is the same pleasure-rewarding neurotransmitter that affects smokers. Just like a drug addict, someone who continually eats chocolate brownies, for instance, raises the threshold of that reward, which means that it gradually takes more and more brownies to regain that initial pleasure. Rather than suppress our desire for any food, we need to re-educate our palates to desire more nutrient-rich food that will fill us up and to shift our focus from using food as a reward.

The third is that our bodies have nutritional requirements that must be met. No amount of willpower will convince a body that is starving for protein that it doesn't need it. That body will just continue demanding protein, or whatever else it needs. The danger is that we often can't tell that the body wants protein. All we know is that it wants something. When we eat a lot of the wrong thing, we end up gaining weight and still are hungry for the nutrition our body needs. An example of this happened when we had a friend over to our house for dinner. She is an avid runner and cyclist. We fixed a chicken stir-fry. Our friend wasn't a vegetarian, but also believed in eating very little meat and never ate red meat. She had four helpings of the stir-fry, purposely choosing servings with lots of chicken. She was a little embarrassed and confused as to why she was eating so much. Her body needed the protein.

What to take away

- Fad diets are quick fixes with false promises. To maintain the weight we want, we need to learn to eat healthily and proportionately.
- Fad diets upset our metabolism. Losing weight slowly maintains a steady metabolism.
- Fad diets cause us to lose weight quickly but not effectively.
- Losing weight slowly will help to keep it off and give us time to refocus our reward system.

3. THE DEADLY TRIAD OF DENIAL

If you really want to do something, you'll find a way; if you don't, you'll find an excuse.

— Frank Banks

Consuming food and beverages is one way our culture provides entertainment and rewards us. It is easy to absorb ourselves in the enjoyment of this form of entertainment and lose track of the pounds we accumulate. When we become aware of the damage that years of indulgence have done, we become angry and frustrated with ourselves and then use food to medicate and deaden our negative feelings. Thus we get even bigger. When we try to confront our behavior, we feel shame and embarrassment and then deny our condition in an effort to hide our shame and anger. Our heavier bodies are harder to move, so we become increasingly sedentary. This vicious cycle is what I call the deadly triad of denial, anger, and shame. Unless we break this cycle and come out of denial, we continue to get bigger and heavier.

It is critical to understand this deadly triad or we won't be able to lose weight and change our condition. All diets, all diet books, and all weight loss programs will fail if we don't understand this. People who are overweight suffer from shame and anger, which puts them into a state of denial. Denial of their unhealthy condition is easier than facing a multitude of fears regarding the possibility of failure or the embarrassment of trying to work out in a public place. It is okay to feel fear but it is not okay to let fear limit your growth.

> *This vicious cycle is what I call the deadly triad of denial, anger, and shame.*

Negative emotions become a breeding ground for anger and resentment. Overweight people are angry with themselves for being too heavy and they often resent anyone that does not have such a problem. They are also frustrated because they really want to be healthy and look better, but just don't have the knowledge and skills to get there. I remember once having lunch with an overweight friend who was frustrated because she wanted to eat better and lose weight, but she didn't know how. We went to a buffet that served whole, natural foods. She tried to put together a plate of food that was balanced, but she had no idea what to eat or why, so she was clearly upset. Once I explained what macronutrients are and gave examples, she was able to navigate through her choices. Knowledge is power.

People who are overweight suffer from the deadly triad of denial, denying their condition, their feelings of shame, and their fear of ridicule and other what-ifs. These emotions feed on each other, making change difficult. To break the cycle, we need to come to terms with how we deny being trapped in the cycle.

Why do we need to understand that we are in denial of our health, fitness, and weight problems in order to succeed with our weight-loss goals?

> *To break the cycle, we need to come to terms with how we deny being trapped in the cycle.*

Until we recognize and confront the problem, the problem cannot be solved. As long as we are able to delude ourselves that there isn't a problem, or we shift the blame for the problem, or we ignore the problem, there is no reason for us to make difficult lifestyle changes. Even though about 67% of Americans are overweight/obese, when questioned in a recent survey, nine out of 10 people recognized when others were overweight but only four out of 10 recognized when they themselves were overweight. Even when people were shown that their height and weight placed them in the overweight category, half of them still insisted their weight was normal. Dr. James Reilly, a gastric-bypass surgeon from Ireland, says that every obese patient who comes in for surgery appears to be oblivious to the fact that they are obese. With a little prodding, some will admit to being "a little heavy."

On a personal note, my husband and I have a friend who weighs nearly 400 pounds. However, if the subject of weight should come up, she will say, "I have a small weight problem, nothing serious." One of my family members was told by his doctor that he was obese. His reaction? He found a new doctor! The reason for this widespread self-deception is largely human nature. As humans, we are afraid of failure and of the unknown, so we deny the unpalatable and the uncomfortable in order to avoid the difficult perceived lifestyle changes needed to solve the problem.

Some people actually get a pay-off from being overweight/obese. They don't see it that way and are not able to articulate it as such, but

> *Some people actually get a payoff from being overweight.*

the payoff is real and creates a barrier against losing weight. For some people, the payoff is avoiding the fear and responsibilities of intimacy and relationships. For others, it can be as simple as avoiding household chores because their excess weight makes it too hard. In my profession I see people using weight as an excuse to not try more demanding types of exercise classes or work out with more intensity. They can tell their friends and family that they work out even though they don't make any physical changes. In their minds, they are absolved of trying more or going harder since they are already "working out" despite little or no changes. Identifying and understanding our motivation to stay heavy can help us find motivation to lose weight.

How do we learn to overcome our fear of failure and denial so that we are able to become fit and lose weight? First, understand that not wanting to perform the work of becoming fit is normal for most of us. It is human nature to want to avoid work. We make devices to make our workload easier. We have remote controls for our TVs so we don't have to get up to change the channel. We have riding lawn mowers so we don't have to push a mower. We use cars so we don't have to walk. The Segway, a motorized device, can be used to carry us in a standing position for short distances, so we don't have to walk even short distances.

Unfortunately most of us equate exercise with work rather than fun. Just observe people at a health club as they drive around looking for the closest parking place to the door, only to run on a treadmill or take a cycling class. At the club where I work, a patron suggested that the management arrange a shuttle service or valet service so people wouldn't have so far to walk from the parking lot! They don't want to do any extra work even though it all helps in losing weight and staying fit.

We stay in denial by engaging in shortsighted habits. We don't always buy things we need; we buy things we want. We don't order foods we know are good for us; we order foods we want. If it happens that we buy or order food that we want and that is also good for us, it's often just a coincidence.

If we are in denial about our weight and fitness level, we will not do anything to change our lifestyle until choices are forced on us. For example, people who are limited in

When we realize things have gone too far, for too long, and there may be no way back, we finally react.

their movement due to their weight have limited choices of where they can go and what they can do. After neglecting important self-maintenance to prevent disease in the first place, people end up with limited choices when they develop a chronic condition or disease. If the condition is terminal, it is too late and there are no choices. Rather than take charge of an outcome, we simply react to whatever happens to us. The situation has control of us; we don't have control of the situation. Simply put, it reaches the "uh-oh, it's too late" stage. When we realize things have gone too far, for too long, and there may be no way back, we finally react. Most of us know someone who quit smoking only after being diagnosed with cancer or emphysema. On the other hand, if we are motivated to confront our health concerns and change our lifestyle, we will have control of our choices far into the future.

I know people who have literally eaten themselves into type II diabetes. When confronted with the diagnosis, only then will they try to manage their diet and their blood sugar. However, damage has already been done to the pancreas, eyes, and the cardiovascular system.

Let me give you an example of denial in action. My husband and I were having lunch at a restaurant that offers a buffet. We saw a very heavy man in his 30s, walking with difficulty as he visited the dessert station over and over and over. I noticed that the lower parts of his legs were reddish and dark, with large darker splotches on them, an indication of very poor blood circulation or how the legs of a person with advanced or untreated type II diabetes look.

If not treated, the next step may be amputation. Yet this man continues to place his health at great risk despite his obvious condition, even though he is a husband and father with people who depend on him.

Many of us don't recognize our own mortality and we tend to take our daily existence for granted. When we make unhealthy choices for ourselves, we are also making unhealthy choices for our spouses, children, family, friends, and coworkers. We are seeing the first generation for whom eating out or

> *When we make unhealthy choices for ourselves, we are also making unhealthy choices for our spouses, children, family, friends, and coworkers.*

ordering in has become as natural as walking. By the time we realize that the condition of our health affects how we live, with whom we live, and where we live, and that we are indeed mortal, it is often too late.

The next chapter will teach how to recognize some of the ways we remain in denial by sabotaging our own efforts to make better lifestyle changes. Any time we find our-

> *If we don't come to terms with denial, the rest of this book is meaningless.*

selves saying "yeah but…" or "I already know that…" we are reinforcing denial and limiting our choices. If we don't come to terms with denial, the rest of this book is meaningless. The first part of solving a problem is acknowledging and confronting it.

What to take away

- Denial is hard to see in ourselves, but easy to see in others.
- Before a behavior can be changed, it must first be identified and described.
- Denial can be frightening, emotionally painful, and thus hard to overcome, but overcoming denial is very much worth it.

4. TYPES OF DENIAL

There are no shortcuts to any place worth going.
— Beverly Sills

Ninety-nine percent of failures come from people who have the habit of making excuses.
— George Washington

Research shows that 90% of people make excuses for not making lifestyle changes such as adopting a healthier way of eating and exercising even though 93% of people would like to be healthier and fit.[2] We have all used denial over the course of our lifetime. Webster's says that denial is *"a refusal to admit the truth or reality…a psychological defense mechanism in which confrontation with a personal problem or with reality is avoided by denying the existence of the problem or reality."*

I have witnessed many times during my career, people who ask how to lose weight and become healthy. I reply, eat less, eat better,

> Denial keeps us in a vicious circle of the deadly triad.

and move more. Almost 100% of the time they respond with "I know, but what else can I do?" Mental health experts agree that denial serves a temporary valuable service to those who need to survive in very difficult circumstances such as prisoners of war or victims of abuse, where the reality is so grim that blocking it helps survival. However, denial that involves not admitting unhealthy lifestyle habits and having trouble admitting the truth and its consequences, including gaining excess weight keeps us in a vicious circle of the deadly triad. Let's look at some of the denial myths that keep us from making lifestyle changes.

MYTH: It's not my fault. I am a victim.
Many people who want to lose weight and become fit are unable to reach their goal because they think like a victim instead of an achiever. Victims don't have control over their choices because they have

abdicated that power to someone or something else. Victims react to situations; they are not proactive and in control of the situation. Time and time again, overweight people are featured on TV programs crying about how poorly they have been treated and how they continue to be disrespected; they act like victims. One TV program followed a man who had become housebound due to his weight.[3] He had been admitted into an expensive weight-loss program at a famous hospital that specialized in treating obesity and he needed to be transported there. Since he weighed over 700 pounds, it took many people plus the removal of part of the outside doorframe to get him out of the house and into the ambulance.

Instead of being grateful for the help being offered to him, he complained that the United States could put people on the moon but could not get him out of his house without attracting national attention and embarrassing him. Let's break this thinking down: he had obviously agreed to be on a TV program and he knew he would be seen by millions of people, so isn't it a little late to be embarrassed? Furthermore, if your neighbor's house were surrounded by vans and TV cameras sporting a nationally known broadcasting logo, wouldn't that be enough to attract attention?

In spite of all the help that was being made available, much of which others did for him, this person was still feeling sorry for himself and thinking like a victim. This mental attitude ultimately prevented him from succeeding in losing weight to become healthy.

Overweight people are seen on TV programs complaining about how they are teased, embarrassed, and discriminated against because

People are discriminated against for many reasons.

of their size. This is true. It does happen. It is rude and disrespectful to behave this way towards overweight people. People are discriminated against for many reasons, including race, religion, sexual orientation, and weight. However, if someone doesn't like you, it is really their problem. If you want to lose weight, you must think like an achiever and become proactive. A grossly overweight person is going to attract attention in the gym or anywhere else for that matter. That's reality and, unfortunately, that is one of the consequences of being overweight. Once you accept that fact, you also accept that you can be proactive and take charge of your health. The outcome will be achieving your goal.

Overweight people may also show "victim" thinking by complaining that they become uncomfortable when they are stared at in fast-food places and other restaurants. Staring is rude, childish

As humans, we are fascinated with people who willingly do something that has a negative impact on their lives.

behavior but it happens. The reason people stare is because we all, including the overweight person, know that eating too much, especially eating calorie-laden, non-nutritious food, will hurt our health. Yet there they are, hurting themselves. The same thing happens to people who smoke, especially young people. Everyone knows smoking is bad for us, yet people do it. As humans, we are fascinated with people who willingly do something that has a negative impact on their lives.

Feeling sorry for ourselves and trying to eat the feeling away only makes the problem worse. People who are successful at losing weight and getting fit are those who understand they are in control of their lifestyle, that their choices made them unhealthy, and that they can choose to be in control of the behaviors that will reverse their situation. Once this barrier is overcome, a feeling of empowerment takes over and the goal of becoming healthy becomes a reality.

Some of the attention an overweight person gets in the gym can be positive. Seeing a person take on a personal commitment and take the necessary means to achieve it is often an inspiration to others around them. I have seen this happen at the facility where I work. Many fitness clubs now offer special, specific classes or programs for people who are too overweight to comfortably take a fast-paced, high-intensity class. Often such people are put on treadmills, use light hand-weights, and are guided through a workout program by an instructor or personal trainer. They are out in full view of other club patrons. Instead of being shunned, these participants are cheered on by other club members. This produces a feeling of achievement and inspiration for all.

Unfortunately, people who are overweight are often victims of well-meaning but enabling friends and family who sabotage the overweight person's environment. Let's take an extreme case. We all know about people who are so heavy they are bedridden and housebound. They can't move or walk, yet they continue to eat and gain weight. One study showed that immobilized people who were between 600-900 pounds consumed 10,000-15,000 calories per day or enough calories to sustain a normal-weight person for five days. How were they getting the food? Their friends and family were giving it to them. Rather than confront the problem, the enablers give in to the demands of the obese for more food.

Not only must we come to terms with our denial, our family and friends need to look at modifying their actions as well, so our personal environment can support our plans for a significant lifestyle change.

> *Not only must we come to terms with our denial, our family and friends need to look at their actions as well.*

MYTH: Big is beautiful.

Another concept that supports denial is to believe in a philosophy such as "Big is Beautiful." This is where a person insists that they are just fine, no matter what size they are. Many people who are severely overweight will admit they are large but claim they are also beautiful and that therefore there is nothing wrong. While good self-esteem is important, it should not be used as an excuse to maintain an unhealthy body or weight. Overweight people can be outwardly attractive but it does not hide that inside, they are not healthy.

A person who is very overweight can dress well to enhance their assets or diminish flaws but this is mostly just window dressing. There is nothing attractive about watching a person walking with difficulty because their weight puts too much pressure on their knees and hips. There is nothing sensual in listening to a well-dressed, well-groomed, and very heavy person gasping because they can barely walk up a flight of stairs.

Star Jones is a well-known celebrity and was a co-host on the TV show "The View." During most of her time with the show, she was obese. When the subject of weight came up, she would insist that at her size she was beautiful and also healthy, even though she could be heard wheezing over her microphone.

A woman on another TV program[4] I saw claimed that even though she weighed more than 500 pounds, she was healthy. Since she believed this, she was not motivated to change her lifestyle. Due to her enormous weight, she suffered from lymphedema, a condition where the body's extremities (arms and legs) collect excessive amounts of fluid, producing rolls and pockets of flesh.

The skin in such areas often breaks down, oozes, is prone to infection, and can give off a putrid smell. She suffered as well from diabetes and elevated blood pressure. Yet she believed she was "healthy" and "beautiful." While it was good to see she had a positive self-image, this person chose to use this positive self-image to continue her denial of her health problems rather than to change her lifestyle.

On the extreme side, one woman, Donna Simpson, weighs over 600 lbs and wants to be 1000 lbs. She spends $750 on food a week, has diabetes, can't manage her personal hygiene herself, and has lymphedema, yet she claims she is normal, beautiful, and healthy.

In a fat-acceptance blog a person wrote, "It may not be healthy if you are really grossly overweight…but if you are portly, or plumpish or a little cuddlier, than others it is not any more of a death sentence than for those that smoke." I'm not making this stuff up! If this isn't denial, I don't know what is.

An attractive person, no matter what their age, radiates good health. Overweight people show their health problems in how they move, breathe, and appear. Being attractive comes down to being healthy; it is not based on a bias against people who are too heavy.

> An attractive person, no matter what their age, radiates good health.

One reason a fit person radiates good health is their balanced hormones. When a person maintains a balanced diet and proper weight and muscle tone through exercise, their hormones stay balanced and help to enhance their health in many ways and this is reflected in their appearance. When women become obese, they often take on masculine traits such as facial hair on their cheeks, chin, and neck.

While overweight women's unbalanced hormones tend to give them masculine features, men who become overweight tend to display more feminine traits, most commonly large breasts. The slang term for these is "man boobs" but the technical term is gynecomastia. In Britain, Dr. Christian Duncan has performed many liposuction operations on teenage boys to reduce the breast tissue in their chest. What was once a rare procedure has become more and more commonplace as people continue to become overweight/obese.[5]

Another feature among men who are overweight is a softer, fleshier, less muscular appearance of the chest, stomach, back, and arms. Some overweight men have less facial hair and softer facial skin and features.

When proper nutrition is neglected, it shows in a person's skin, nails, eyes, hair, gait, and, of course, their size.

When proper nutrition is neglected, it shows in a person's skin, nails, eyes, hair, gait, and, of course, their size. In addition, being unhealthy increases a person's risk for heart disease, cancer, diabetes, and arthritis.

Sexual attraction is based on visual attraction. Attraction is defined by symmetry in the shape of a person's eyes, nose, mouth, cheeks, chin, and forehead and how these features line up on the face and what their proportions are. The symmetry of our bodies also refers to the proportion of the head to the lengths of other parts of the body. These would be the arms, legs, torso, hands, and feet. Symmetry also is about the proportions of the chest, waist, and hips to each other and to the extremities. Being overweight puts these proportions out of symmetry and creates a distorted appearance. Therefore, to insist that "Big is Beautiful" not only supports denial of an unhealthy body, it also denies eons of human evolution.

Throughout human history, the human form has been manipulated to enhance, exaggerate, or diminish certain body parts and segments in the name of beauty, but always within the parameters of set ratios and measurements. For example, in the Middle Ages, a woman who had a rounded, distended abdomen was considered attractive because she looked newly pregnant and thus fertile. However, there was still symmetry between her breasts, hips, and waist. Despite the different ways the human form has been manipulated throughout history, the attention to symmetry has remained constant.

MYTH: Thin is in.

The most common health risk these days is being overweight, but it is important to also look at the other side of the coin. Being too thin is unhealthy, too. Models starve to

Being too thin is unhealthy, too.

achieve a thin look, but there is really nothing attractive about a person who is so frail and thin that every movement appears likely to break them in two. There is nothing sensual about a person who looks like a living mummy or a walking coat hanger because they lack muscle tone. Very thin people, like overweight people, can make themselves outwardly attractive but they cannot completely hide their unhealthy insides.

People who are too thin display a lack of health and radiance, and therefore can be unattractive even when well dressed and groomed.

Just as overweight people have health problems that make them less attractive, underweight people run similar risks. When women are very underweight, they lose their menstrual periods, bone mass, and the fat padding that supports their breasts, face, and buttocks. Their hair, skin, and nails become brittle, thin, and dull. All of this gives them an aged and haggard appearance. They no longer have a radiant appearance or a curvy, sensuous figure. Men who are anorexic suffer bone and supportive fat loss, along with unhealthy skin, hair, and nails just as anorexic women do, giving them an aged, stooped stance as well as a skeletal appearance.

Denial is a huge factor in anorexia. The person's body always appears to be too large. Serious health risks are ignored in an attempt to achieve a "perfect" figure. Professional help from a therapist is usually required before changes can be made.

□ ■ □ ■ □

Those are the big myths that lead to denial. Now let's look at some of the other myths that support denial or reinforce denial.

MYTH: I'm not fat/unhealthy, but you are.

WHY WE THINK THAT: It is easier to see in others what we cannot see in ourselves. In fact, we often see easily in others the very thing that bothers us most about ourselves.

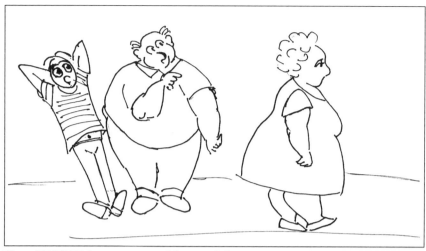

Now THERE is someone with a weight problem.

THE FACTS: It is easy to draw attention to others who do not eat a healthy diet or exercise, but we often are in denial about what and how much we eat or exercise ourselves. Dr. David Schutt of Thomason Medstat, a data collection and analysis company, found that more than three quarters of obese Americans claim they have healthy eating and exercise habits.[6] As mentioned earlier, he discovered that nine out of 10 people can see that other Americans are overweight, but only four out of 10 can see that they are overweight. When people in the study were shown how their weight and height placed them in the overweight category, half considered themselves to be "just right."

The responses from obese people about healthy living habits paralleled those of thinner respondents. For example, 19% of obese people claimed they read, understood, and relied on nutritional labels, compared to 24% of people of normal weight who said the same thing. Around 40% of obese people and 30% of normal-weight people admitted to eating everything served to them at restaurants. Around 40% of obese people claimed they do vigorous exercise at least three times a week, as did the normal-weight responders. Regardless of whether we are obese, overweight, normal-weight, or underweight, the conclusion is that we all seem to believe we engage in the same "healthy" eating and exercise habits and are "just fine." If we believe we are "just fine," why would we change?

MYTH: As long as I eat good foods, calories don't count.

WHY WE THINK THAT: The media and countless numbers of diet books have all claimed that if we just follow diet "XYZ," we can eat all we want and don't have to count calories. It is human nature to want to take the easy way out.

THE FACTS: If you take nothing else away from this book, please take this: ALL CALORIES COUNT! It doesn't matter if we eat 4,000 calories a day of whole foods,

If you take nothing else away from this book, please take this: ALL CALORIES COUNT!

fruits, and vegetables or 4,000 calories of Twinkies and pizza. If we don't burn off those 4,000 calories, we will store what we don't burn. Calories are real and to successfully lose weight, we have to burn more calories than we take in, no matter what diet we are following. If we eat three pounds of food, where does that three pounds go? We will use and process some of it, and the rest of the calories will be stored in our body, not in a rental unit!

Despite this, diet authors commonly advise us to forget about counting calories. No wonder most people fail in their weight-loss efforts! This disregard for the impact of calories began in the 1980s with the philosophy of a low-fat, high-carbohydrate diet. Health authorities led millions to believe that dietary fat was the cause of obesity. We were encouraged to slim down by cutting out fat and replacing it with carbohydrates. The rationale for this claim was that a gram of dietary fat contained over twice as many calories as a gram of protein or carbohydrate. Has the low-fat philosophy worked? As we now know, the anti-fat/low-fat campaign didn't just fail, it backfired!

We became convinced that, as long as we kept our fat intake low, we could eat as many carbohydrate-rich foods as we wanted and not gain weight. The result of this mis-

As we now know, the anti-fat/low-fat campaign didn't just fail, it backfired!

guided diet philosophy can be observed all around us. Decades of low-fat consumption has helped produce the fattest, most obese, and most diabetic population the world has ever seen.

As we began to understand that the low-fat diet was a failure, we turned towards its opposite, the low-carbohydrate diet. Beginning in the late 1990s, a string of best-selling

No matter what "diet" a person is on, 12 servings of anything is too much!

low-carbohydrate diet books came out. All had a common theme. As long as we stayed away from carbohydrates, a high-protein, high-fat diet would allow us to eat as much as we wanted without putting on weight.

The authors claimed the real diet villains were carbohydrates because an abundance of carbohydrates will encourage our bodies to produce excess insulin. They enthusiastically urged their readers to forget about counting calories and instead focus on cutting carbohydrates. This faulty advice led Isabelle Leota and her husband Sui Amaama to believe they could consume all they wanted in protein and fat at a local buffet called the Chuck-A-Rama. Even though a buffet implies all you can eat, Sui was on his 12th serving of prime rib when he and his wife were asked to leave the buffet for consuming too much meat.[7] One serving of prime rib is 470 calories so 12 servings is 5,640 calories, or nearly three times the average total daily calorie intake. No matter what "diet" a person is on, 12 servings of anything is too much! Calories matter!

Time and time again, tightly controlled metabolic studies have shown no difference in the rate of weight loss in people who are on high- or low-carbohydrate diets with the same number of calories. Nor do these diets have differing effects on metabolic rates. If we want to lose weight, we must consume fewer calories than we expend. We must create a calorie deficit, either by reducing our caloric intake, increasing our physical activity level, or, ideally, both. All the fancy diet plans in the world won't change this inescapable fact.

MYTH: I really don't eat that much.

WHY WE THINK THAT: Most of us don't know how much we really eat because eating is more than just a refueling mission; it is also a social and emotional activity. We tend to pay more attention to our companions or surrounding environment than to how much is on our plate or how much is going into our mouth.

THE FACTS: We routinely underestimate the amount we consume each day and at each meal. Studies show that 80% of us underestimate how much we eat. Ironi-

> *We routinely underestimate the amount we consume each day and at each meal.*

cally, the heavier we are, the less we think we eat. In conjunction with this, many of us also eat unconsciously throughout the day. One dietician tracked her unconscious eating by writing down each item she ate whenever she went by her coworker's desk. Before looking at her list, she estimated she had eaten only one piece of candy and one cookie. Her results showed she had really eaten four chocolate miniatures, two mints, four shortbread cookies, and three fruit candies for a total of 596 calories. That is one entire meal's worth of calories! Not only was she unaware of how much she ate, she did so without thinking about it.

My husband and I went to our state fair to see some of the entertainment. Many people go to the fair to eat as their form of entertainment. We watched two shows over a period of 3½ hours. An overweight couple who sat in front of us ate the entire time. They ate as a form of entertainment, not for nutrition. This is because eating and drinking is fun! It is easy to get lost in the enjoyment of eating and drinking and lose track of the accumulating pounds. Doing anything to excess isn't good. My husband says it is like watching people chain-smoke, only they are chain-eating.

Consuming tiny bits of snacks lying around the house or office adds up to lots of calories. Polishing off the last bites of food in our cabinets and refrigerator also adds lots of unnecessary calories. For example, drinking that last little bit of orange juice in the carton rather than putting it back in the refrigerator adds up to 26 calories. The two tablespoons of granola left in the box comes to 64 calories. At work, the "small" sample of cake in the break room is 73 calories. Two small mints to keep your breath fresh add up to 20 calories. Those small pieces of chocolate from your coworker's jar give you 25 calories each and nobody ever takes just one! That handful of trail mix in the bowl on the table is another 105 calories. After work, the grocery store's cheese-and-cracker sample is another 55 calories. At home, the two tablespoons taken for a taste test while cooking macaroni and cheese are 54 calories, and then the ¼-cup serving for dinner is another 108 calories. All of this adds up to an extra 555 calories that we typically overlook.

We serve ourselves with utensils that hold much more than a serving. In an experiment, two groups of women were told to serve themselves ice cream using one of two different-sized spoons. Each group served themselves one scoop as one serving, even though one group used a bigger serving spoon.

Consuming tiny bits of snacks lying around the house or office adds up to lots of calories.

Since 1977 portion sizes in restaurants and at home have increased dramatically from what they used to be. We need only three ounces of meat at a meal and that is a serving about the size of a deck of cards. A serving of cereal, rice, pasta, mashed potatoes, or ice cream should be about the size of half a baseball. A serving of cheese should be about the size of a nine-volt battery or three dominoes. One tablespoon of butter, mayonnaise, or oil should be no more than the size or volume of the tip of one's thumb. A tablespoon of salad dressing or peanut butter should be only the size of half a ping-pong ball. When eating out, share that huge entrée with a friend or family member, or put half away in a take-home container before even starting to eat.

Since 1977 portion sizes in restaurants and at home have increased dramatically.

MYTH: My hormones are to blame for my weight and I can't do anything about it.

WHY WE THINK THAT: We would like to shift the blame for our weight problem to something we think is out of our control so we don't have to be responsible.

THE FACTS: The two most common hormonal abnormalities that cause weight gain are hypothyroidism and Cushing's syndrome. Symptoms of hypothyroidism (too

Most obesity is caused by lifestyle choices but it never hurts to rule out other reasons with a medical evaluation.

little thyroid hormone) are fatigue, swelling of the face and eyes, dry skin, lack of sweating, slow, hoarse speech, poor memory, and intolerance to the cold. Cushing's syndrome is caused by an excess of the hormone cortisol. People with Cushing's tend to accumulate fat in the face and upper body while their arms and legs remain slender. A medical check-up and blood work can eliminate these relatively rare hormone problems as the cause of any unwanted weight gain. Most obesity is caused by lifestyle choices but it never hurts to rule out other reasons with a medical evaluation.

MYTH: Cooking nutritious meals takes too long and is too expensive.

WHY WE THINK THAT: Let's call it what it really is. We are either bad cooks, we don't like to cook, or we are just lazy. Just so you know, I'm not picking on the reader since I qualify for at least two out of the three excuses on any given day! However, these excuses can be overcome. Most of us would rather have someone else do the work of getting the groceries, figuring out the recipe, preparing the food, and serving it. We also have been convinced that buying prepared foods, which are often full of chemicals and preservatives, is better and cheaper.

THE FACTS: In the time it takes to select a restaurant, drive there, which consumes gasoline, *Going out for fast food is not fast!* park, wait to be seated, wait for a server, wait for the order, eat, and drive home, consuming more gasoline, we could have made a wholesome meal of seasonal foods, cleaned up the kitchen, and had time to relax and do other things. Ordering fast food for delivery takes just as long and is just as costly, if not more costly. Owners of take-out or fast-food restaurants need to make a profit so they can pay their drivers, buy the ingredients, pay for the upkeep of their buildings, and pay their employees and themselves. Those expenses are reflected in what we are charged for the food. In the meantime, we need to pick a place, make a phone call, wait on hold, and then wait for delivery. Going out for fast food is no faster! Again, we must pick a place, get there, find a parking place, wait in line to place the order, find a seat, eat, and then go home, using more gasoline.

If you need more convincing, try this. The next time you plan to have cheap fast food, think about the expense. How much is this meal going to cost you? Now compare that to your favorite expensive food

---
A homemade meal is usually less expensive than "cheap" junk food.

---

that you buy at the store and prepare yourself. My experience is that the homemade meal is usually less expensive than the "cheap" junk food. And it tastes better and is better for you.

MYTH: I may be overweight, but I am fit.

WHY WE THINK THAT: Again, the media has given us permission to think that since some of us are overweight and active, we are fit. We think we have accomplished our goal when, in reality, we are just starting the journey.

THE FACTS: It is certainly better to exercise than not to exercise, especially if overweight. However, being overweight puts pressure on the hip and knee joints, stresses the heart, and increases the risk of acquiring other chronic ailments. Dr. Amy Weinstein, a heart specialist at Boston's Beth Israel Deaconess Medical Center, says that exercise doesn't eliminate the risks of chronic disease and joint problems in the overweight person.[8] Weight still matters.

This Harvard study compared thousands of women over a period of eleven years who were either:[9]

The normal-weight and active women had the lowest risk levels for heart disease, joint problems, and other ailments.

- normal-weight and active
- overweight and active
- obese and active
- normal-weight and inactive
- overweight and inactive
- obese and inactive

The normal-weight and active women had the lowest risk levels for heart disease, joint problems, and other ailments. The overweight and active women's risks were 54% higher than the normal-weight and active women, and the obese and active women were 87% more at risk. Among all the inactive women, those with normal weight had a slightly higher risk than the normal-weight and active women. The overweight and inactive women's risk was 88% more than the normal-weight and active women's, and the obese and inactive women had even higher risk. The conclusion: if a person is overweight/obese yet still active, they remain at substantial risk for heart disease, joint problems, and other chronic ailments. A more realistic way to view being overweight/obese and active is to realize that you are on your way to a healthier lifestyle but not there yet.

Another study involved 5,000 men at the University of North Carolina from 1972-1998.[10] Each man was grouped into two of four categories: fit or unfit, and fat or lean. Those who were unfit and fat faced the greatest health risks. The lean and unfit group also had a shorter lifespan than either of the fit groups. Those who were lean and fit had the least risk. In the group that was fit but fat, exercise helped to promote longevity but did not compensate for the other negative health risks brought on by excess weight.

Let's examine the life of a Japanese Sumo wrestler. Most Sumo wrestlers are over six feet tall and can reach weights close to 800 pounds. Even with these statistics,

Exercise cannot offset all the negative health risks that come with excess weight.

Sumo wrestlers have more muscle, less fat, and better reflexes than inactive people of the same height and weight. But are Sumo wrestlers healthy? The Japanese have the longest life span of any people on earth. Men have a life expectancy of 78.6 years and women have a life expectancy of 85.5 years. Japanese Sumo wrestlers have a life expectancy of less than 60 years or the same life expectancy as someone of the same weight who is not a wrestler.

Sumo wrestlers, including the younger ones, suffer from knee and hip problems that lead to falls during matches. They have sleep apnea, a side effect of being obese, and have heart problems. When Sumo wrestlers retire at the age of 35-40, they must deal with health issues more common among retirees in their 60-70s. These include arthritis, heart disease, and diabetes. Being active when overweight/obese is good but a healthy, manageable weight enhances the benefits of being active.

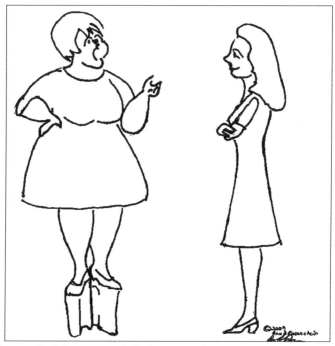

Well, for my height, my weight is normal.

The bottom line: Although exercise will help offset many health risks regardless of whether we are overweight or lean, exercise cannot offset all the negative health risks that come with excess weight.

MYTH: My obesity is inherited.

WHY WE THINK THAT: We all know families that are comprised of heavy parents and heavy children, with heavy aunts, uncles, and cousins. We believe what we see.

THE FACTS: It does seem that there is a genetic link but this is true in only a small number of people. Scientists have been working hard to identify genes that have the potential to make us fat. One such gene that has been identified is a variant of a gene called FTO. People who had two copies of the variant gene were more likely to be heavier than those who had only one copy. Those with one copy of the variant were heavier than those who had no copies of the gene. However, having or not having the gene didn't automatically determine a person's weight. In the study to find the gene, there were people who had two copies of the gene but were not overweight, and there were people who didn't have the gene at all and were overweight. The presence of the gene seems to only confer a predisposition to being overweight and is only one of many influences on a person's weight. As a result, most experts agree that while genes may have a part to play, genes don't explain the recent rapid increase in obesity in the Western world. Researchers believe that while we might inherit "fat" genes from our parents, we also "inherit" their bad habits, such as poor diet and lack of exercise. These poor lifestyle habits have a more important impact on our weight than our genes.

MYTH: My set point is what it is.

WHY WE THINK THAT: We believe that we have a set point that determines how much we weigh and that it cannot be altered.

THE FACTS: If we really all had a set point, we would not be able to gain or lose weight. The set-point theory suggests that while fat cells can grow or shrink, they prefer to stay a constant size. When we overeat, we fill up our existing fat cells. If we continue to overeat, we create additional, new fat cells. According to the theory, this resets the set point. When a person dramatically reduces their intake of food to the point of becoming anorexic, their fat cells shrink and, if they continue to starve themselves, the fat cells begin to die. To me this is an oxymoron. If a constant can be reset, it is not a constant. Therefore, a set point is not a set point!

MYTH: I am just big boned.

WHY WE THINK THAT: If we have "big bones," then we can carry more weight.

THE FACTS: Some people have smaller frames, but the difference in the mass of the bones of people with larger frames is not so great that they can support excess pounds and unnecessary weight.

> If we can pinch more than an inch around our midsection, we are carrying too much weight.

Regardless of frame size, if we can pinch more than an inch around our midsection, we are carrying too much weight. Frame size can be

Table 2: Wrist measurement and frame size.

Height	Wrist Measurement	Frame
Men Over 5'5"	Less than 6.5"	Small
	6.5"-7.5"	Medium
	Over 7.5"	Large
Women Under 5'2"	Less than 5.5"	Small
	5.5.-5.75"	Medium
	Over 5.75"	Large
Women 5'2"-5'5"	Less than 6"	Small
	6"-6.25"	Medium
	Over 6.25"	Large
Women Over 5'5"	Less than 6.25"	Small
	6.25"-6.5"	Medium
	Over 6.5"	Large

assessed by measuring the distance around the wrist where there is usually little fat and no muscle to add to the measurements. For example, people with wrist measurements less than 5.5" and who are less than 5'2" are considered to have a small frame and those whose wrist is greater than 5.75" are considered to have a large frame.

MYTH: I don't have time to make changes.

WHY WE THINK THAT: Again, let's call it what it is, fear. We are afraid to venture into the unknown, even if it might be better. We fear leaving the comfort of what is familiar, even if what is familiar is unhealthy. It takes effort and concentration to change our behavior. It is normal and okay to be afraid. It is not okay to let fear stifle your choices.

THE FACTS: Everyone already knows that a number of factors contribute to weight gain. It's not just about finding time to exercise, or about choosing healthier foods, it's about a genuine commitment to

If we're not ready to make permanent lifestyle changes, losing weight and becoming fit and healthy will be hard.

making healthy decisions every day regardless of what else is happening in our lives. If we're not ready to make permanent lifestyle changes, losing weight and becoming fit and healthy will be hard. Here are 10 things we need to do in order to get started:

Attitude. If we go on a health kick only to lose weight or look a certain way, we will not lose weight permanently. If we don't see results quickly, we will likely give up. Weight loss and its benefits are great goals, but unless we have something else to motivate us, nothing will keep us going if the scale doesn't budge. It takes time to lose weight, and we have to motivate ourselves in the meantime. Find more reasons to be healthy and lose weight, such as having more energy, getting off medications, not dealing with chronic health problems, or living longer to be around for your children and grandchildren. Those are long-term, worthwhile reasons.

Exercise. If we don't work out consistently enough, it's harder to lose weight, and we don't build muscle tone. While it's possible to lose weight with diet alone, we'll eventually hit a plateau. It's not necessary to spend hours in the gym, killing ourselves with impossible workouts. We only need a reasonable fitness schedule that we can follow each week. It's about being active on a regular basis by finding something we like that we'll continue to do for the rest of our lives, not just for a day here and there.

Diet. Changing the way we eat is another thing we must do for long-lasting weight loss. We need to willingly replace unhealthy foods with healthier choices each day. This might mean:

> *For permanent weight loss, we need to pay attention to what we eat and to make good choices more often than not.*

- Keeping a food journal. And don't lie! The scale will keep you honest.
- Spending more time in the grocery store reading food labels.
- Spending more time preparing meals.
- Saying "no" to extra portions.
- Making informed, conscious choices about *what* we put in our mouth, *when* we put something in our mouth, and *why* we put something in our mouth.

For permanent weight loss, we need to pay attention to what we eat and to make good choices more often than not. A structured diet eventually ends, but healthy eating never stops. There will never be a time when we're done with healthy

> *For permanent weight loss, we need to pay attention to what we eat.*

eating. We might feel like we're sacrificing the good stuff (pizza, fast food, etc.) and that our life won't be fun if we can't have those foods. The good news is we can still have them, but not as often or we can learn to make our own version. As we adopt new ways of eating, we learn to appreciate the taste of whole, nutritious foods and to make negative associations with less nutritious foods. If we are willing to make these changes and spend time planning what and when to eat instead of consuming the most convenient and often fattiest or sweetest food available, we will have made a healthy lifestyle change that results in permanent weight loss.

Lifestyle. If we want a healthy life, we need to be willing to change how we live. That doesn't mean changing everything overnight, just being open to new ways of doing things. Here are a few ideas:

- Daily routines. We may need to get up earlier to prepare lunch or squeeze in a workout. Or we might use part of our lunch hour for exercise, or go for a walk after work instead of watching TV.
- Limits. We might need to set limits on how much TV we watch and how long we sit at the computer. We'll need to pay attention to how much time we spend being sedentary so we can add more movement.
- Our pantry. If we're the kind of person who will eat an entire bag of Doritos or devour an entire bag of cookies, then we don't keep them in the house. If someone brings them home, they must be told to not bring them home again and to relocate them immediately. If we want to be healthy, we need to gradually get rid of those unhealthy foods that we just can't resist.
- Schedule. It's going to be hard to lose weight if we're not willing to change the way we live each day to take time to prepare meals, exercise, and nurture ourselves with sleep. We use busy

schedules as an excuse not to have a healthy lifestyle. If we're not ready to take responsibility for the schedule we've created, it will be hard to lose weight.

Surroundings. Sometimes we can't control the things around us. At work, we may be surrounded by temptations such as doughnuts, vending machines, homemade

If we eat an entire bag of Doritos or cookies, then we don't keep them in the house.

treats, and other bakery goods. This will force us to make choices to stay committed to a healthy lifestyle. At home, surround yourself with things that will support your efforts to get healthy. For some of us this might mean spending some money on home workout equipment, setting up a corner of the house for workout gear, or commandeering the TV a few nights a week to do an exercise video. Some of us do better going to a health club where the workout environment is contagious. Either way, when at home, set up an environment that encourages healthy choices.

Support system. While getting healthy may be something we're doing on our own, it's helpful to have a support system. This includes family members who understand what we're doing and are either willing to participate or help us reach and maintain our goals. If we have a spouse who wants to continue eating the kinds of foods that tempt us, we need to have a plan to deal with this so we can still reach our goals and keep our relationship together. We need to surround ourselves with people who support what we're doing and avoid people who make and/or encourage bad food choices on a daily basis. A workout partner can also provide excellent support.

Spiritual and mental health. For many of us, food represents comfort like a friend we've relied on our whole life to help us deal with emotional problems. Some of us eat out of an emotional need and not because we are hungry. Our cravings are triggered by our association with a particular food and the emotion it evokes. Many of us eat ice cream, bread, or chocolate because as children we were consoled in one way or another with these foods and eating them not only fills us physically, these foods fill an emotional void. One of my overweight clients told me that food was her friend because food never hit her, abandoned her, or called her names. For her, food was the one thing that was constant and dependable. These foods became her friends and we don't just abandon our "friends." A counselor can help with this, or try reading about emotional eating. Be willing to learn why we make the choices we make and confront them.

Some try hypnosis or other behavioral techniques to help overcome emotional cravings. One technique that seems to be effective is

Food was the one thing that was constant and dependable.

EFT. EFT stands for Emotional Freedom Techniques. In randomized study, ninety-six overweight or obese adults were assigned to the EFT treatment. The degree of food craving, perceived power of food, restraint capabilities, and psychological symptoms were assessed before and after a four-week EFT treatment program and at a 12-month follow-up. Paired comparisons between time-points were undertaken using post hoc tests. EFT was associated with a significantly greater improvement in food cravings, the subjective power of food, and craving restraint from pre- to immediately post-test.[11]

If we try to soothe away our emotional pain or depression with comfort foods, it's going to be hard to lose weight. Pinpointing those behaviors and emotions and what drives them is important so we can become aware of what we're doing, why we do it and change the behavior.

Goals. If we set impossible goals, we are guaranteed to fail and when we feel like a constant failure, we can't lose weight. The key is to set reasonable goals for ourselves.

We need to pick goals we know we can achieve so we will be successful.

Those goals are going to be different for each person, depending on our genetics, eating habits, exercise, and metabolism just to name a few. Set up long-term goals, whether to lose weight or compete in a race, and focus on daily or weekly goals. A weekly goal might be to get in three workouts, minimum. We need to pick goals we know we can achieve so we will be successful. The goal can be as big or as small as we like, as long as we can do it.

Flexibility. We hear and read a lot about lifestyle changes, but it's the daily choices that really test us. What happens if we have to work late and can't get to the gym? Or what if we get stuck in traffic or in a snow-storm and miss our fitness class? Any number of things can happen in a day that may upset our schedule. The solution is to be flexible. Be pre-pared for scheduling conflicts by keeping some workout shoes in the car, so you can stop off at the park for a quick walk. Keep some food and water handy, so you can get a snack in before your workout if you get stuck in traffic. Often we skip workouts because something comes up and we simply aren't ready for it or we aren't willing to give ourselves other options. Sometimes we believe if we can't get a full workout in, we should skip it completely. However, something is always better than nothing! Another option is to go on a different day.

Willingness to fail. We will not be perfect every day. Everyone has good days and bad days. On the good days, we'll eat all our fruits and veggies, say no to greasy pizza, and do our workout even though we're tired. On the bad days, we'll wake up late, forget to bring our lunch, have an extra piece of cake at our friend's birthday party, and skip our work-out. The bad days will happen because we're human. The answer is to never give up, even when we mess up. We're not going to fail our overall goal just because we make some mistakes. We need to try to do our best to make good decisions and gradually change.

What to take away

- Denial is very hard to beat. Just remember: if a solution is pre-sented and we respond with "yeah but…" or "I'm different…," we are in denial. Until we come out of denial, the rest of this book won't matter.
- Calories matter! They add up, no two ways about it!
- Every action we take or decision we make is a choice.

5. METABOLISM

I went to the 30th reunion of my preschool. I didn't want to go, because I've put on like a hundred pounds.

— Wendy Liebman

You better cut the pizza in four pieces, because I'm not hungry enough to eat eight.

— Yogi Berra

We are often frustrated because we gain weight as we age. We believe that we gain weight because our metabolism slows down with age. We also believe that thin people have a fast metabolism and overweight people have a slow metabolism.

Before we can debunk these metabolism myths, we have to understand a little about metabolism. Metabolism is the chemical process our body uses to build and destroy tissues. Metabolism releases energy in the form of movement and heat. When we exert our bodies during physical exercise, we speed up our metabolic process and burn more calories. When we are at rest, our metabolic process slows down. We continue to expend calories at rest, only not as many in the same amount of time.

The basic rule of metabolism is a series of math equations. One pound of body fat equals 3,500 calories. To lose a pound a week means subtracting 500 calories a day. This can be best achieved by cutting 250 calories from our diet and burning 250 calories each day through exercise. For many people, this means eliminating one can of soda pop, a bowl of ice cream, or a bag of chips a day. That's the key for most people who successfully lose weight and keep it off.

To lose a pound a week means subtracting 500 calories a day.

Just reducing calories makes it difficult to get the nutrients we need. For long-term success, we need to learn a new way to live, not just a temporary way to diet. Studies with "successful losers" find that they all use similar tactics:

46

- Engage in daily physical activity.
- Reduce overall calorie intake.
- Eat breakfast.
- Monitor weight on a regular basis.
- Maintain a consistent eating pattern.
- Catch "slips" before they turn into larger weight gains.

A generally accepted method to determine whether one is within normal weight limits is to calculate body mass index (BMI), which is closely equivalent to basal metabolic rate (BMR), the number of calories a person burns at rest, which can only be measured under special laboratory conditions. BMI is a number calculated using height and weight and is the same for either sex. The standard BMI categories and numbers according to the World Health Organization are underweight (<18.5), normal weight (18.5-24.9), overweight (25-29.9), class I obesity (30-34.9), class II obesity (35-39.9), class III obesity (>40). Table 3 shows the BMI ranges for selected heights.

Table 3: BMI and its relationship to height and weight.

Height	Healthy	Overweight	Obese I	Obese II
5'3"	105-140 lbs	140-169 lbs	170-225 lbs	225+ lbs
5'6"	115-150 lbs	151-182 lbs	183-240 lbs	240+ lbs
6'0"	136-180 lbs	181-217 lbs	218-290 lbs	290+ lbs

A limitation of the BMI standard is that this measure does not take into account fat versus muscle mass. Since the more lean muscle a person has, the higher their BMR will be, BMI may misclassify some people. Nonetheless, it remains the most generally accepted and commonly used method for weight classification.

MYTH: Metabolism slows with age.
WHY WE THINK THAT: Most people we know gain weight as they age, so it is easy to assume that age and weight gain go together like eggs and bacon.

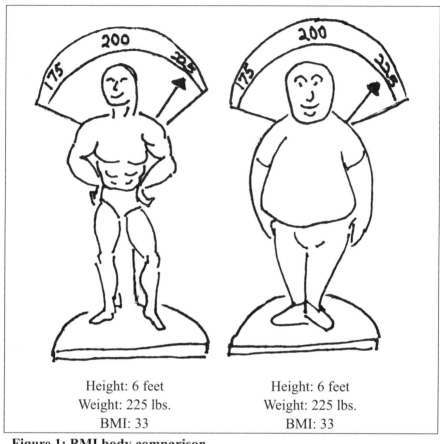

Height: 6 feet	Height: 6 feet
Weight: 225 lbs.	Weight: 225 lbs.
BMI: 33	BMI: 33

Figure 1: BMI body comparison

THE FACTS: There is no biological reason to gain weight as we age, yet we do. This is because we tend to reduce our activity levels as we age, thus the number of calories we burn drops and our lean muscle mass decreases. Less lean muscle mass means we have a lower metabolic demand, so we use fewer calories to maintain the same weight. When we don't exercise, our muscles atrophy (shrink) and they don't need or burn as many calories. However, when we don't exercise, we tend to consume the same amount of food or more food, which leads us to the conclusion that our metabolism must have slowed down.

While it is true that our metabolism is slower, what is not true is that it slows down with age. A given amount of food, exercise, and muscle mass produces the same results at any age. If you want to lose weight, eat less, exercise more, and build up your muscles.

> *A given amount of food, exercise, and muscle mass produces the same results at any age.*

MYTH: Women gain weight after menopause.

WHY WE THINK THAT: As women age and go through menopause, their hormones change. Since most people we know seem to gain weight with age and women seem to gain weight after the onset of menopause, it is easy to blame hormonal changes for the weight gain.

THE FACTS: While hormones can be blamed for a lot of things, from acne to PMS, excess weight is more likely caused by inactivity rather than hormone changes. Study after study has found that women who exercise regularly and vigorously well into middle age maintain their sensuous figures. Weight charts imply that as we get older, we need to limit our calories simply to maintain our weight. These charts don't differentiate between active and inactive people; instead they assume that advancing age, instead of inactivity, accounts for our increased weight.

MYTH: You are born with either a slow or a fast metabolism.

WHY WE THINK THAT: Most of us eat the same way we did when we were younger, but we don't move as much, as fast, or as often as we did when we were young. Since we don't think we are eating more and we don't like to admit we are becoming less active, we would rather blame our metabolism.

THE FACTS: No matter who you are or how old you are, one pound of muscle burns three times as many calories as one pound of fat. This is a metabolic constant. If

> *One of the beauties of losing weight with exercise is that is gets easier as you increase your muscle mass.*

two people weigh the same, but one has more fat mass than muscle mass, that person is going to burn fewer calories than the person who has more

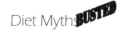

muscle mass than fat mass. One of the beauties of losing weight with exercise is that is gets easier as you increase your muscle mass.

MYTH: Heavy people have a slower metabolism than thin people.
WHY WE THINK THAT: It is human nature to believe what we see. If a person is overweight yet claims to eat a modest amount, then logic and our eyes tell us they must have a slow metabolism.

THE FACTS: The average 5'5", 120-pound woman has a BMR of about 1,300 calories a day. That means it takes 1,300 calories a day just to keep all of her bodily functions operating at rest. Another 5'5" woman who weighs 220 pounds will have a BMR of about 1,680 calories a day. At first glance it appears the heavier woman has a faster metabolism than the thin woman. The reality is the heavier woman has more overall mass to maintain, so her BMR is higher, but her metabolism is not faster. Herein lies the paradox: as a person loses weight and their body mass decreases, their overall BMR will decrease. However, as muscle mass increases with exercise and fat stores decrease, the lean muscle mass will burn three times as many calories as fat. If the 220-pound woman loses 100 pounds and develops a higher ratio of muscle to fat, then her total BMR will be higher in relation to her new, smaller size.

Along with BMR, a person's daily activity level needs to be considered. For example, if our 120-pound, 5'5" woman works in an office for eight hours and is sedentary most of the day, she may only

> *As muscle mass increases with exercise and fat stores decrease, the lean muscle mass will burn three times as many calories as fat.*

need a total daily intake of 1,800 calories to sustain her weight. This assumes that she only needs 500 extra calories per day over her BMR. This is an unrealistic expectation for most people because most people eat at least 2,000 calories a day. However, if this same woman increases her daily activity level by, for example, biking or walking to work, walking at lunch, and taking the stairs rather than using the elevator, she may need closer to a total of 2,200 calories a day to maintain her weight. This tends to give the illusion that she has a fast metabolism since she will consume more calories but maintain her same size. In reality, because she

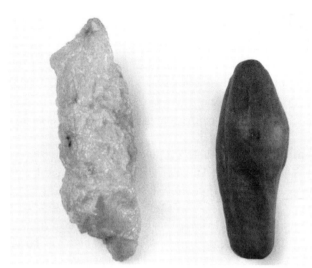

Figure 2: Five pounds of fat next to five pounds of muscle. Although they weigh the same, the fat is larger.

has increased her activity level, she has increased her lean muscle mass and decreased her fat mass, thus increasing her BMR.

MYTH: Eating small meals through the day is better than one or two meals a day.

WHY WE THINK THAT: We have been told or have read numerous times that eating many small meals will keep us full and will help us burn more calories as well as prevent us from overeating.

THE FACTS: How many calories we burn is determined by our BMR, the rate at which we burn calories at rest. When we have more muscle mass compared to our fat

Constant grazing is one way to lose track of how much we eat and can lead to overeating.

mass, we burn more calories, no matter how many meals we eat or how often. When we eat at regular times and more than a few times a day, we hopefully will not overeat since we won't feel starved. However, constant grazing is one way to lose track of how much we eat and can lead to overeating. Waiting until we are ravenous sets us up to gobble down the first foods we see and we may eat so fast that we will become overfull before our brain can signal our body that we are satisfied.

The bottom line: Eat three sensible meals a day, with a couple of balanced snacks when needed, but don't sweat it if you can only get a couple of meals in. If your lifestyle includes a couple of days where eating at regular intervals is difficult, carry some wholesome snacks with you to hold you over till you can relax at a meal. As long as we have lots of muscle mass, we will burn calories at a fairly high and constant rate.

MYTH: Skipping meals can help me lose weight.

WHY WE THINK THAT: This certainly sounds plausible: if we skip a meal, we are cutting down on calories; if we cut down on calories, we will lose weight.

THE FACTS: People who think skipping a meal will lead to weight loss do not understand how our bodies work. If we skip a meal, our

If we skip a meal, our bodies will think that we are starving.

bodies will think that we are starving and will therefore hoard our energy reserves to compensate. This is why we are often tired and lethargic when we haven't eaten in a while. Then, we are so hungry by the time we do eat that we tend to overeat at the next meal. Skipping a meal and then eating too much at the next meal often means that we have a higher total caloric intake than if we just ate more frequently throughout the day. A better approach is to eat smaller, more frequent, healthy meals and snacks to keep our blood sugar balanced.

Studies show that people who skip breakfast and eat fewer times during the day tend to be heavier than people who eat a healthy breakfast and eat four or five times

Breakfast skippers compensate for those missed calories by eating more throughout the day.

a day. Breakfast skippers actually compensate for those missed calories by eating more throughout the day. People who regularly eat breakfast tend to have better luck losing weight and keeping it off.

A good breakfast is a bowl of low-sugar, high-fiber cereal with milk, banana, whole-wheat toast and jam and peanut butter or other nut butter, and, if you wish, tea or coffee. A great breakfast is a hardboiled egg and a small bowl of slow-cooked oatmeal topped with berries, walnuts, raisins, flaxseeds, or sunflower seeds, and, if you wish, coffee or tea.

Not only do we need to eat breakfast, we need to start the day off with the right food: If we grab only a doughnut or muffin, we will be ravenous before lunch because of a rapid rise and fall in blood sugar. However, if we cut our calories too far or below 1,200 a day we'll end up with a double whammy. We will decrease our muscle mass and that will lower our BMR. A lower BMR means we burn fewer calories at rest. To get the most out of the calories we eat, we need to choose whole foods, such as produce, fresh meat and fish, and whole grains, that are as close to their natural state as possible. They have a higher "nutrient density" than refined foods because they pack more vitamins and minerals into fewer calories. An occasional skipped meal is not going to change our metabolism, but it shouldn't become our norm.

MYTH: Calories eaten after 8:00 PM will be automatically stored as fat.

WHY WE BELIEVE THAT: Most of us are inactive in the evening, so we believe any food eaten after we relax will not be actively used.

THE FACTS: This myth is no truer than the notion that the moon is made of green cheese. The fact is that if we eat more calories than our bodies burn in a day, the excess

> *There is no connection between calories and the clock. It does not matter what time of day we eat.*

calories will be stored as fat. Whether we consume calories during "Good Morning America" or "The Tonight Show" doesn't matter. There is no connection between calories and the clock. It does not matter what time of day we eat. What matters is what we eat, how much we eat, and how much physical activity we get during the whole day. No matter when we eat, our body will store unused calories as fat. For example, I teach a 1-hour fitness class two nights a week and my husband teaches a 1½-hour class one night a week, so my husband and I end up having dinner around 8:00 PM or later more than one night a week. After those classes, we need to refuel!

The bottom line: Let hunger guide you. If you come home late and are hungry, eat a small, wholesome, balanced meal. However, if you have eaten a fulfilling, satisfying dinner but now sit in front of the TV at 9 or 10 PM with a bowl of ice cream, that may mean you are eating to fill an emotional need and not for hunger. Eat a nutritionally balanced breakfast. This will prevent a junk-food splurge later in the day. No matter when you eat, create a calorie deficit if you want to lose weight.

MYTH: Combining certain foods should be avoided.
WHY WE THINK THAT: There are plenty of crash diets and fad diets based on the belief that our digestive system can't handle a combination of foods or nutrients. Carbohydrates and proteins are often said to "clash," leading to digestive problems and weight gain.

THE FACTS: The opposite is often true. Foods eaten together can help the digestive system. For example, the vitamin C in an orange or green pepper can increase iron absorption from a meal of chicken or beef. Very few foods are purely carbohydrate or purely protein; most are a mixture of both. Our digestive system contains corrosive enzymes and hydrochloric acid that can eat a hole right through a tabletop! Therefore our digestive system is perfectly capable of breaking down the foods we eat.

There are some exceptions to this, though, so the myth is sometimes true. One important one is that calcium found in dairy products, for example, will reduce the absorption of iron.

> *Our digestive system contains corrosive enzymes and hydrochloric acid that can eat a hole right through a tabletop!*

MYTH: There are foods that cause weight loss.
WHY WE THINK THAT: There is a long-standing, widespread belief that celery, cabbage, and lettuce take more calories to digest than they produce, so the action of eating them gives us a calorie deficit. We also believe that grapefruit is so low in calories that we burn more calories to process it. We also think that since caffeine makes us hyper and raises our blood pressure, it will burn a significant number of calories.

THE FACTS: There are no foods that cause our bodies to burn more calories than we take in. In fact, it just goes against nature. We eat food to sustain us, not to diminish us.

Dietary fiber comes the closest to fulfilling this fantasy because it provides a feeling of "fullness" from bulk, not from calories. Caffeine may speed up our heart rate, which may burn a few more calories, but this lasts for a short time and burns an insignificant amount, so does not affect our weight. The grapefruit diet requires you to eat half a grapefruit before every meal to reap the benefits of the fruit's so-called fat-burning enzymes, but the existence of these enzymes has never been proven. Furthermore, the diet limits calorie intake to fewer than 800 calories a day, which is why we lose weight. It has nothing to do with grapefruit! We could eat just as many lemons, achieve the same results, and call it the Lemon Diet. Grapefruit has no fat, is low in calories and sodium, and is packed with vitamin C. But that very low total-calorie intake, along with deficits in protein, fiber, and several important vitamins and minerals, makes this diet dangerous. Similarly, proponents of the cabbage-soup diet report feeling lightheaded and weak because the diet is too low in protein, vitamins, and complex carbohydrates. You may lose weight, but you'll be too malnourished to enjoy it. You will fart all the time, making you unpleasant to be around, and the weight loss won't last unless you continue to eat only cabbage soup. Not a good return on your investment!

MYTH: Diet pills enhance metabolism and contribute to weight loss.

WHY WE THINK THAT: Unfortunately, we live in a pill-popping society. We are constantly looking for the magic pill that will give us the body we want without doing the hard work it really takes. Just watch cable TV on Saturday or Sunday morning.

THE FACTS: Initially after taking diet pills we will lose weight due to the lowered requirements of food and calories, but in the long

Taking a pill does not teach us how to control our weight.

run we will gain more weight back. Taking a pill does not teach us how to control our weight through proper nutrition and lifestyle changes. Diet pills also present a danger, as they are not regulated by the FDA, contain questionable ingredients, and can become habit-forming.

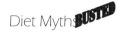

MYTH: Natural or herbal weight-loss products are safe and effective.

WHY WE THINK THAT: We think if something is "natural" or "herbal," it must be safe.

THE FACTS: A weight-loss product that claims to be "natural" or "herbal" is not necessarily safe. These products are usually not scientifically tested to prove that they are safe or that they work. For example, herbal products containing ephedra have caused serious health problems and even death. Newer products that claim to be ephedra-free are not necessarily danger-free, because they may contain ingredients similar to ephedra or may have other ingredients that are dangerous even though we may not know it yet. Remember, just because it is natural doesn't mean it is safe or beneficial. Cow pies are naturally produced by cows but you wouldn't want to eat one, even with ice cream!

> *Just because it is natural doesn't mean it is safe.*

What to take away

- Advancing age and changes in hormones don't automatically mean we will gain weight.
- A lack of physical activity causes us to gain weight, and there are no foods that burn excess fat.
- Our metabolism is based on how much muscle mass we have in relation to how much fat mass we have. The more lean muscle we have versus fat, the more calories we need to consume to maintain our weight.
- How much we need to eat is based on our muscle-to-fat ratio, not the time of day or night or the combination of foods.
- Muscle burns calories at a constant rate, which is three times higher than the rate that fat burns calories.

6. MACRONUTRIENTS

> You really are what you put into your body. You can't run on
> fumes. You don't put a lousy gasoline in a top-quality car.
> — Martina Navratilova

My intent is to keep this book and this information as simple and as understandable as possible. I am only going to tell you what you MUST know to manage your diet and to dispel the myths and misinformation surrounding food and diet. Before we can dispel myths and misinformation, we need to understand macronutrients and how the macronutrients in food are metabolized by our bodies. You need to understand the macronutrients in the foods you eat and how they affect your body and your lifestyle.

Our bodies are fueled with food in a way similar to how a car is fueled with gasoline. Our bodies metabolize food, turn it into energy, and use that energy to perform bodily functions and to recover from everyday wear and tear. Our lifestyle and food choices dictate how efficient our metabolic processes are.

After we have eaten, the body uses oxygen to convert food into energy. The nutrients that provide energy come from macronutrients called carbohydrates, proteins, and fats. They are either used to fuel the body or they are stored as fat. Any waste will be expelled in the form of carbon dioxide, water, or solid byproduct.

Carbohydrates are the body's main source of energy and are broken down quickly into sugars that are stored in muscle and the liver as

> *Carbohydrates are the body's main source of energy.*

glycogen. The body's muscle cells can only store a certain amount of glycogen at any given time. Excess sugar is stored as fat.

Carbohydrates are the major source of energy for the body because, of all the nutrients, they are most easily converted to glucose, a kind of sugar, which is the body's preferred fuel. Carbohydrates are converted in the digestive tract to glucose, which is distributed by the liver through

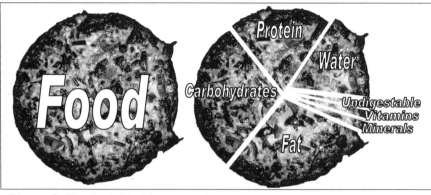

Figure 3: Food divided into nutrient classes.

the bloodstream for cells throughout the body to use as energy. Once immediate energy needs are satisfied, the remaining glucose is either converted to glycogen, a temporary source of readily available energy stored in the liver and muscles, or converted into fatty acids by the liver and stored in fat cells throughout the body.

Proteins are used by the body to build and maintain the body's cells and tissues. As with carbohydrates, the cells can only store a certain amount. Excess protein is stored as

> *Proteins are used by the body to build and maintain the body's cells and tissues.*

fat. Protein is broken down into amino acids in the stomach and small intestine, then distributed by the liver through the bloodstream to cells throughout the body for a variety of uses including cell formation and repair. Surplus amino acids remain circulating in the bloodstream. This surplus is either converted into a type of simple sugar and used as energy or, like surplus carbohydrate, is converted into fatty acids and stored in fat cells.

Fat is the most efficient, densest, longest lasting source of fuel. Our bodies use fat to guard against starvation. Unlike carbohydrates

> *Our bodies use fat to guard against starvation.*

and protein, the body's cells can store an almost infinite amount of fat, regardless of whether the original source was excess carbohydrates,

Table 4: The macronutrients and their functions.

Macronutrient	Function	Calorie Content
Carbohydrate	Provide quick energy	4 calories/gram
Protein	Build and maintain tissue	4 calories/gram
Fat	Store energy, provide long-term energy, and protect cells	9 calories/gram

proteins, or fats. Our bodies typically store enough glycogen for 90 minutes of fuel expenditure and enough fat for 119 hours in the muscle.

Dietary fat is broken down into fatty acids and glycerol by the stomach and small intestine. These materials are then distributed, in the form of triglycerides, by the lymphatic system and bloodstream to cells throughout the body for a variety of specialized uses or, if there are insufficient carbohydrates in the body, for energy. Since dietary fat cannot be converted into protein and only about five percent, the glycerol, is convertible into glucose, a significant amount ends up being stored as body fat if it is not used as fuel.

Good lifestyle habits teach the body to burn fuel with greater efficiency. When the body is operating efficiently, it will use greater

Good lifestyle habits teach the body to burn fuel with greater efficiency.

amounts of oxygen to convert more food into useable fuel and will burn fat first. Less carbon dioxide is produced and less food is stored as fat.

Macronutrients can be found in whole foods and in "junk foods." The problem with junk foods is that they produce *free radicals* along with the macronutrients. A free radical is any molecule floating freely and ready to attack our cell structures. Junk foods do not provide nutrients that are able to oppose this. When the cell structure is attacked, the healthy cell is changed and will either die or replicate with this new change included as a mutation. This creates a burden for our immune system. Free radicals are also found in pollutants. Since there are plenty of free radicals all around, why choose to ingest them?

Antioxidants are molecules that can safely intercept or interact with free radicals to stop them before a chain reaction damages vital cell structures.

In the human body, free radicals are believed to cause tissue damage at the cellular level by causing damage to our DNA, mitochondria, and cell membranes. This tissue damage has been associated with premature aging, cancer, heart disease, and other human ailments. These conditions are aggravated by things such as excessive alcohol intake, smoking, various chemical exposures, and ingestion of nutrient-deficient foods. To prevent free radicals causing damage, the body uses a defense system of antioxidants that are found in whole, unprocessed foods.

An antioxidant is a molecule that is capable of donating its electrons without becoming unstable and thus does not rob the healthy cells of their electrons.

> *An antioxidant is a molecule that is capable of donating its electrons without becoming unstable.*

The human body uses energy to power its muscles and fuel the millions of chemical and biological reactions that take place within our body every day. This energy comes from the specific molecules we consume in our diet: water, protein, fats, and carbohydrates. These nutrients are digested and/or absorbed by the body in the gastrointestinal tract, then processed and absorbed by the rest of the digestive system in different ways.

If energy is suddenly needed, the body can convert fat into energy. The body first uses up its glycogen reserves, and then it converts body fat to energy by a catabolic process called lipolysis. During lipolysis, triglycerides are converted into fatty acids and glycerol. The fatty acids are then transported through the bloodstream to tissues for use as energy or, along with glycerol, to the liver for further processing.

Fat cells are specialized cells that synthesize and store globules of fat. This fat comes from the dietary fat we eat or is made by the body from surplus carbohydrates and proteins in our diet. Fat tissue is mainly located just under the skin, although fat deposits are also found between the muscles, in the abdomen, and around the heart and other organs. The location of fat deposits is largely determined by genetic inheritance. We can't decide where we store fat or influence which area the body burns fat from for energy purposes. This is why there is no way to "spot-reduce."

One way many of us become fat is by eating more calories than we burn off in activity. Along with a lack of exercise, we live in a culture that emphasizes "value-for-money food portions" in the form of buffets. We have "super-sizing" steadily increasing serving sizes in restaurants and an almost constant introduction of new, tasty, high-calorie foods and energy drinks. This often leads to overconsumption and often to obesity.

What to take away

- We need all the macronutrients, preferably in their most natural form.
- We need to keep our intake of fats, proteins, and carbohydrates balanced. More of a good thing isn't a good thing.
- Excess calories from any source will cause weight gain.

7. CARBOHYDRATES

Anyone who eats three meals a day should understand why cookbooks outsell sex books three to one.

— L.M. Boyd

I tried every diet in the book. I tried some that weren't in the book. I tried eating the book. It tasted better than most of the diets.

— Dolly Parton

Carbohydrates, along with fats and protein, are one of the three main elements of food known as the macronutrients. Carbohydrates are organic compounds consisting mainly of sugars, starches, and fiber. Plants make carbohydrates during photosynthesis and store them in the form of saccharides (fiber) and sugars. These carbohydrates can be used for energy by the body. However, if they aren't used in short order, they're stored in the liver and muscles as glycogen and what can't be stored there is stored as fat.

From our body's standpoint, carbohydrates are sugars. Except for the fiber in carbohydrates, which we cannot break down into glucose, all carbohydrates, whether simple or complex, are broken down into sugars.

Carbohydrates are organic compounds consisting mainly of sugars, starches, and fiber.

The only question is how quickly do the sugars make it into our bloodstreams? Does the carbohydrate cause a rapid, high rise in blood glucose, or does it break down over a longer period of time, thus allowing blood sugar to rise slowly and not peak as high?

Carbohydrates cause blood sugar levels to rise. When it rises quickly, we are infused with a rush of energy that leaves us almost as quickly as it came, leaving us hungry after just a short time. If our blood sugar rises slowly and steadily, we have energy for a longer period of time and have longer stretches between hunger pangs.

Unfortunately, most of the carbohydrates we consume are simple and refined. The misconception we often have is that starches, which are complex carbohydrates, are broken down slowly in our bodies. This is true only if they are consumed in their whole and unrefined state, not if the starches are the ones in most processed foods we find in the grocery store. Food manufacturers begin the process of breaking carbohydrates down for us by grinding grains into flour, refining grains, puffing rice by removing the husks, which extracts the nutrition, and then flavoring them by adding sugar. Whole-wheat flour, which we commonly believe is natural and whole, is actually refined and almost as high in sugars as white flour.

Non-starchy vegetables, legumes, and low-sugar fruits are nutritious sources of carbohydrates and include most of the best sources of

Legumes are a good addition to our diet.

phytonutrients, the organic components that help the body fight off disease, as well as being superior sources of vitamins, minerals, and fiber. Legumes are a good addition to our diet because they contain carbohydrates that are slowly digested. When choosing grains, eat whole (intact) grains, such as basmati rice, barley, quinoa, and bulgur. Whole grains are broken down more slowly than if they are ground into flour.

The Glycemic Index

The glycemic index is a measure of how a food affects blood sugar levels. It was developed over 20 years ago in 1981 by researchers

There are many reasons why the glycemic index is not very practical.

Dr. David Jenkins and Thomas Wolever of the University of Toronto[12] to show that not all carbohydrates raise blood sugar levels by the same amount. For example, the research showed that potatoes raise blood sugar quicker than fruit, while legumes, such as lentils, beans, and peanuts, raise blood sugar more slowly than either fruit or potatoes. Different fruits also raise blood sugar levels at different rates.

There are many reasons why the glycemic index is not very practical. The glycemic index is based on the results of eating only one food at a

time. However, when we eat our food at a meal, we combine carbohydrates with proteins and fats on one plate, and even in one forkful. Combining foods changes the glycemic value of the entire meal, and that
changes the rate of glucose absorption. This is why a processed candy
bar might rank lower on the glycemic index than a whole-food item, such
as an apple, but that doesn't mean the candy bar is nutritionally better
than an apple!

Other factors that affect the glycemic index:

- The types of starch in foods can affect their rate of digestion.
  Complex starches digest more slowly than simple starches.
- Physical form of the food. For example, the seed coating around
  legumes acts as a barrier to digestive enzymes, slowing the rate
  of digestion and lowering the glycemic index.
- The portion size of the food. One carrot has a low glycemic
  index but five carrots have a higher index.
- The ripeness of the fruit or vegetable. The riper, the higher the
  index.
- Whether the food is cooked or raw. Raw food has a lower index
  than cooked.
- How quickly or slowly we eat. The slower we eat, the slower we
  digest, and the lower the index.
- Our current blood sugar level. When blood sugar is high, stom-
  ach emptying is delayed; when the glucose level is low, stomach
  emptying is faster.
- If we take medication for diabetes, and, if so, how much.
- The time of our last medication, the time of day we ate, and/or
  the length of time since our last meal.
- Our level of physical activity.
- Our stress level and health status.

Eating only foods with a low
glycemic index limits food choices.
An important guideline for healthy
eating is to eat a variety of foods, in
moderation, throughout the day. The

*The complexity of the glycemic
index makes it difficult to apply it to
our daily eating.*

complexity of the glycemic index makes it difficult to apply it to our daily eating. The glycemic index is useful in helping to understand the basic impact a food has on our system, but that is all. We need to think bigger by considering the whole meal.

How We Spike Our Blood Sugar Levels

Here is a typical scenario for how consuming too many carbohydrates can elevate blood sugar levels and why carbs get such a bad reputation. We typically eat a breakfast unbalanced in macronutrients and full of carbohydrates: cold cereal, bagels, doughnuts, muffins, pancakes, waffles, and toast with jelly, washed down with fruit juice. All these carbohydrates are high in sugars and cause our blood sugar to spike. Then, just a few hours later, our blood sugar plunges in what is known as "the morning crash" produced by *hypoglycemia*, a state of low blood sugar. This can also happen if we skip breakfast. Symptoms of hypoglycemia are cravings for sweets or starches, anxiety, irritability, fatigue, and feeling mentally dull. To offset this feeling, we grab a cup of coffee to wake ourselves up, giving us the "tired-wired" feeling.

Next comes lunch. We often just grab something quick and convenient to make our hunger and cravings go away. If we are "dieting," we may have just a salad, which, to

Food items from the vending machines are all full of refined carbohydrates.

our body, may be just sugar since some salads are composed almost entirely of carbohydrates. We might have fast food, which is laden with dense, nutritionally poor calories that bring on the "afternoon slump" making us feel compelled to take a nap, but we can't fall asleep at our desk! So we reach for more coffee and a quick pick-me-up like a candy bar, a bag of chips, or something else from the vending machines. Food items from the vending machines are all full of refined carbohydrates, drive our blood sugar up, and rob our body of enzymes, minerals, and vitamins, especially B vitamins.

Then there is dinner. We come home from work, undernourished, overfed, and tired, so who wants to cook? Instead, we eat out or order in a convenient high-carb, high-fat meal like pizza, thus keeping the vicious cycle going.

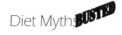

Let's take a look at the myths.

MYTH: Starches are fattening and should be limited.

WHY WE THINK THAT: Fads come and go, and right now it is popular to blame starchy carbohydrates for making us fat.

FACT: Starches are carbohydrates, but they don't make us fat, excess calories from any of the macronutrients make us fat. Often,

> *Excess calories from any of the macronutrients make us fat*

those excess calories are found in the sugar contained in many carbohydrates, especially those that are processed and have had their fiber removed and replaced with added sugar. Starches that are complex carbohydrates are an important source of energy. Examples of these foods are whole-grain bread, unrefined rice, unrefined pasta, whole-grain cereals, beans, fruits, and vegetables. All these foods are low in fat and calories and provide the body with valuable nutrition as well as keeping the colon clean and healthy because of their high fiber content.

When starches are refined and altered from their natural state or are combined with other processed ingredients, they become a problem. Potatoes in their natural state are a great source of nutrition, but potato chips or French fries are not. Pasta cooked until just firm (*al dente)* is a more complex starch than pasta cooked until soft and mushy. Whole-grain pasta has more fiber and is more filling than processed pasta. Raw fruit and vegetables are more nutritious per calorie than those packed in sugar syrups. Like any other food, carbohydrates should be eaten in moderation as part of a balanced diet that includes the other macronutrients.

MYTH: To lose weight, avoid carbohydrates and eat a high-protein diet.

WHY WE BELIEVE THAT: We have bought into the mass media's claim that carbohydrates are the enemy of our weight-loss attempts and programs.

THE FACTS: This myth is partially true. People who are obese may want to decrease their intake of carbohydrates for a short period of time, but they should not avoid them totally. The message conveyed by many low-carbohydrate diets is that consuming lots of carbohydrates promotes too much insulin production, leading to insulin resistance, which, in turn, results in weight gain. We believe that if we deny ourselves carbohydrates, our body will begin to burn glycogen, our body's stored form of carbohydrate, for energy. When our body burns glycogen, water is released, so the initial weight loss we experience is from water, not stored fat. The truth is that, just like other diets, low-carb diets are calorie-restricted. Those eating a low-carb diet may consume only 1,000-1,400 calories a day compared to the average intake of 1,800-2,200 calories a day that we may need. It doesn't matter if we eat a high- or low-carb diet if we only consume 1,000-1,400 calories a day because, if we decrease our caloric intake to less than what is needed to maintain our current activity level, we will lose weight.

Many of the myths and misconceptions about low-carb diets will be discussed in more detail in Chapter 16. Those who condemn low-carbohydrate diets portray people on them as eating an unhealthy diet

Many low-carb diets focus on nutritious, healthy food.

lacking vegetables and fruits, guzzling whipping cream, eating bacon-wrapped steaks, incurring heart disease, and going down a dangerous road to poor health. The truth is that many low-carb diets focus on nutritious, healthy food. Research into reducing carbohydrate intake continues to show more and more positive results.

MYTH: Multigrain foods are always made with whole grains.

WHY WE BELIEVE THAT: Any multigrain bread or pasta sounds so healthy that we think it must be made with whole grains. That is exactly what advertisers want us to believe.

THE FACTS: The only way to know this for sure is to see if the word "whole" is in front of the name of every grain in the ingredient list. "Multigrain" only means the product was made with several grains rather than one. We can't assume that whole or unrefined grains were used. The same is true for "7-grain" or "cracked wheat." Even breads and cereals that say "made with whole grain" often contain only a small percentage of whole grains. So in reality, multigrain foods are made with multiple types of grains that are likely to be in a refined state, thus drastically reducing their nutritional value.

"One hundred percent whole-wheat" breads are made with wheat flour but are generally nothing more than slightly improved versions of enriched white bread. This is because the whole-wheat bread is

> Even breads and cereals that say "made with whole grain" often contain only a small percentage of whole grains.

made with processed flour from wheat sources and is still nutritionally weak. To make sure we are getting real whole-wheat bread, the first ingredient listed must be "whole wheat," "whole-wheat flour," or "stone-ground whole-wheat flour." Any of these means that the grain was ground in its whole state that includes the kernel, bran, and stalks.

Beware of the words "bleached" and "enriched" in the list of ingredients. "Bleached" and "enriched" mean that, since the grain used to make the bread was processed, the natural nutrition was removed and then the nutrition was chemically replaced. Stay away from breads that have "high-fructose corn syrup" or "HFCS" and "hydrogenated fats" or "partially hydrogenated fats" in the list of ingredients.

MYTH: Brown-grain products are whole-grain products.

WHY WE THINK THAT: The color brown makes us think of "dirt" and the color white makes us think of "clean," so a brown food must have come straight from the ground, and must therefore be "natural" and "whole."

THE FACTS: Brown dyes and additives can make foods appear to be whole-grain when they're not. Read the labels carefully to be sure a food contains whole-grain ingredients.

MYTH: Bagels are better than doughnuts.

WHY WE THINK THAT: Bagels are found in the health food aisle and may appear to be made with whole grains. Doughnuts are

> One bagel is equivalent to seven servings (slices) of bread.

found in the bakery section along with sweet, gooey foods such as birthday cakes, cookies, and pies.

THE FACTS: A bagel contains around 300 calories by itself and up to 700 calories when eaten with cream cheese. The flour used to make a bagel is refined, just as in a doughnut, and very quickly becomes sugar once it is in our system. A plain sugar doughnut contains around 150-200 calories. One slice of bread is one one-ounce serving. Since a bagel is often seven ounces, one bagel is equivalent to seven servings (slices) of bread.

MYTH: Eating fiber causes problems if you have irritable bowel syndrome (IBS).

WHY WE THINK THAT: Most of us don't know the difference between the two basic types of fiber in our diet. If a person with IBS consumes insoluble fiber, they may have trouble, and then they think all fiber will cause them problems.

FACT: There are two kinds of fiber: soluble and insoluble. Insoluble fiber can cause problems in IBS sufferers but soluble fiber is easily handled by everyone's bowel and helps prevent constipation. People with IBS should consult their physician about how much insoluble fiber is safe for them to consume. Soluble fiber delays the time it takes food to move through the intestine, while insoluble fiber speeds up this process, which helps prevent constipation in people who do not have IBS. Soluble fiber helps to lower serum cholesterol, while insoluble fiber has no effect on cholesterol. Insoluble fiber will keep the colon healthy and clean, which helps to prevent colon cancer.

Good sources of soluble fiber are flaxseeds, legumes, grains, such as oats, barley, and rye, certain vegetables, such as broccoli, carrots,

Soluble fiber helps to lower serum cholesterol.

Brussels sprouts, and artichokes, some fruits, such as apples, pears, raspberries, blackberries, strawberries, bananas, plums, and prunes, and root vegetables, such as parsnips, rutabagas, potatoes, sweet potatoes, and beets. Insoluble fiber is found in whole wheat and in most fruits and vegetables.

MYTH: Potatoes and bread are fattening.

WHY WE THINK THAT: The low-carb craze has blamed these two foods for most of our weight gain, especially since these two foods are so prominent on fast-food menus.

THE FACTS: Starchy foods like potatoes and breads contain complex carbs used to fuel every part of the body from the brain to the muscles. In their whole, unrefined, and natural state, potatoes are a great source of nutrients without a lot of calories. Whole-grain breads provide high-quality nutrients without a lot of calories.

If the breads or potatoes are refined and processed, have other refined, non-nutritious fillers added to them, or are deep-fried or heavily

In themselves, potatoes and bread are not fattening.

buttered, their calorie content can double, triple, or even quadruple and their nutritional value decreases as well. In themselves, potatoes and bread are not fattening. How they are prepared or processed makes all the difference.

MYTH: Sweet potatoes are better than white potatoes.

WHY WE THINK THAT: We believe this because most of us eat highly processed versions of white potatoes, such as French fries or potato chips.

FACTS: For starters, sweet potatoes and yams are not potatoes at all. Yams are related to the lily and grass families while sweet potatoes are part of the morning-glory family. Sweet potatoes and yams are generally baked and eaten whole. Eaten whole, they retain their nutrients and digest more slowly so our insulin levels do not spike. White potatoes and sweet potatoes have complementary nutritional differences; one is not better than the other. Sweet potatoes have more soluble fiber and vitamin A, while white potatoes have more iron, magnesium, and potassium. The type of potato is less important than the form in which the potato is consumed: whole or processed.

MYTH: All popcorn is healthy.

WHY WE THINK THAT: Read any diet book; we find popcorn on the list of acceptable snack foods.

FACTS: It depends on how the popcorn is prepared and how much is consumed. Air-popped popcorn is the best choice since it isn't smothered in butter and salt. Even though butter is a perfectly acceptable food, cutting down on any unnecessary calories helps if a person is watching their calorie intake. Microwave popcorn and movie theater popcorn are typically loaded with trans fats and salt, thus packed with large quantities of unhealthy calories and sodium.

MYTH: Dried fruit is not as healthy as fresh fruit.
WHY WE THINK THAT: Canned, frozen, and dried foods are safe and convenient, but some of us think if it's canned, preserved, or frozen, it's inferior.

FACTS: Fruit is part of a balanced, healthy diet. It doesn't matter if the fruit is fresh, frozen, or dried. If the fruit is canned in heavy syrup,

Fruit is part of a balanced, healthy diet.

there will be added calories from the sugar syrup, so look for fruit that is packed in water. Often, canned fruit is peeled, so it loses some of its fiber. Juices, even 100% pure, are already processed, so it is easy to consume a lot of calories in a short amount of time. Although juices still have vitamins and nutrients, they have none of the fiber found in fresh fruit.

Dried fruits are real fruit, but the action of dehydrating the fruit reduces the size of the fruit so it becomes easy to eat a lot. A dried raisin has the same calorie content as a plump grape but, due to their size, one handful of raisins is more fruit than one handful of grapes. Even more troubling is the fact that Sun-Maid, Ocean Spray and other companies add sugar to their dried fruit, making their products closer to candy than Mother Nature's original intention. An alternative is to dry your own fruit.

Of course, it's not always possible to purchase fresh fruits and vegetables directly from the farm but, even so, fruits and vegetables are best if eaten soon after picking. Fresh fruits and vegetables straight from the produce aisle are usually best if we eat them soon after purchase. Seasonal changes will affect which type of produce we purchase since out-of-season fresh fruits and vegetables can be quite expensive.

An alternative to purchasing fresh fruits and vegetables is to try canned or frozen. Frozen produce is nutritionally comparable to fresh. Flash-frozen produce tends to retain nutrients better than fresh produce over time, since fresh produce

> *An alternative to purchasing fresh fruits and vegetables is to try canned or frozen.*

continues to age during transportation and while sitting on the shelf before getting to our table. Canned produce loses some vitamins and minerals during the heating process. However, at least three vegetables benefit from the canning process and are actually higher in healthful phytochemicals than their fresh versions: corn, carrots, and tomatoes. Another benefit of frozen and canned produce is their longer shelf life, so they can be kept on hand for quick additions to meals. If purchasing canned or frozen produce, make sure the label says they do not contain added salt and sugars. Avoid fruits in heavy syrup.

MYTH: Yogurt with fruit on the bottom is low in calories and healthy.

WHY WE THINK THAT: Fruit is healthy and yogurt is healthy. Fruit is low in calories and yogurt is low in calories. So the combination of these two low-calorie foods creates a food low in calories.

THE FACTS: Those over-sweetened yogurt cups contain as much sugar as a soft drink. The sugar comes directly from the "fruit," which is swimming in high-

> *Those over-sweetened yogurt cups contain as much sugar as a soft drink.*

fructose corn syrup. Yogurt and fruit can be a great way to start our day, but we can do it best by mixing a cup of plain yogurt with a half cup of fresh or frozen mixed berries. Store-bought "fruit on the bottom" yogurt contains 190 calories and 30 grams of sugar. Plain yogurt with fresh fruit has 110 calories and only 15 grams of sugar, which is from the healthier, natural fructose in the fresh fruit.

What to take away

- Carbohydrates are an important macronutrient.

- We can only use so much carbohydrate at a time. Excess carbohydrates are stored as fat.
- Too many carbs, especially processed and refined carbs, spike our insulin and cause hormonal imbalance.
- It is more important to eat at least five servings of fruits and vegetables each day than it is to worry about how they made it to our plate.
- When choosing starches, pick those that are still in their whole state, such as whole potatoes, whole sweet potatoes and yams, and whole-grain breads, rice, cereals and pasta.
- Carbohydrates are a good source of vitamins and nutrients as long as they are not refined and processed.

8. PROTEIN

Man does not live by bread alone...
— Matthew 4:4

Red meat is not bad for you. Now blue-green meat, that's bad for you!
— Tommy Smothers

Protein is one of the three major classes of foods called macronutrients. The other two are fats and carbohydrates. Proteins are made up of amino acids, also known as the "building blocks of life." We get protein primarily from poultry, beef, lamb, pork, and other animal products, including almost anything that swims, walks, or flies, as well as dairy products such as eggs, milk, and cheese. Protein also comes from plant sources such as legumes, seeds, and nuts.

Protein furnishes the raw materials our bodies need to make muscles, organs, hair, neurotransmitters, and enzymes. Proteins are used to

Protein furnishes the raw materials our bodies need.

make and repair our cells. Specifically, protein is used in the formation of new protoplasm, the technical term for the goo inside our cells. Antibodies and hormones are also made of proteins. Finally, our body can break down protein for energy, but only if all carbohydrate and fat is gone. Unlike carbohydrates or fats, which usually provide us with energy, proteins typically are used to build parts of the cell. When excess protein is eaten, the extra protein can be broken down into energy-yielding compounds. However, if the energy is not used promptly, excess protein turns to fat. Protein prevents us from starving. According to research done at the University of Sydney, the human body is programmed to keep eating until it gets enough protein. Simply put, without protein we would die.[13]

Foods that contain all the necessary amino acids are considered complete proteins. Most animal foods are complete proteins. Some plant proteins are complete proteins, such as soybean products and tofu.

Incomplete proteins are those containing small amounts of one or more essential amino acids. Most plant foods, such as legumes, nuts, seeds, grains, and vegetables, contain incomplete proteins. Although plant proteins are incomplete, it is possible to get all the essential amino acids by eating a combination of plant proteins. For example, peanut butter is low in the amino acid methionine but high in the amino acids lysine and isoleucine. Bread has a lot of methionine, but it lacks lysine and isoleucine. So a peanut butter sandwich is a meal with a complete protein.

Foods from animal sources are complete proteins because they contain all the essential amino acids. In most diets, a combination of plant and animal protein is recommended.

A lack of protein will lead to a weak body that will be unable to fight against disease.

A lack of protein will lead to a weak body that will be unable to fight against disease. Certain diets can result in the body not getting enough protein. We may get enough calories for our energy needs, but we may not get all of the essential amino acids.

Let's look at the myths.

MYTH: It is necessary to consume extra protein to build muscle mass.

WHY WE THINK THAT: Weight lifters, bodybuilders, and trainers tell us we need extra protein, and we believe them. Often they have protein supplements they want to sell.

THE FACTS: Consuming extra protein does nothing to build up muscle mass unless you are also engaged in significant weight training at the same time, which the average person isn't. Actually, the opposite is closer to the truth. If you build more muscle through exercise, then you will need a little more protein than the average person. Bodybuilders often subscribe to the "if a little is good, then more is better" philosophy, and gorge themselves with protein-rich foods and supplements. One popular bodybuilder claims to ingest as much as 1,000 grams of protein a day! To effectively build muscle, we need to lift enough weight to challenge our muscles beyond their normal resistance levels. With all the misunderstandings about protein diets, it is easy to believe that protein is the best fuel for building muscle, but since muscles need calories to work, all three types of nutrients are needed. Unfortunately, the body only has the capacity to utilize a limited amount of protein. Once the saturation point is reached, additional protein is of no use to the body, and it is either used as energy or converted into triglycerides and stored as fat.

By itself, protein has no effect on muscular gains. Contrary to claims made by various manufacturers, protein powders and supplements aren't magic formulas for building muscle. We can't expect to simply consume a protein drink, or eat a thick steak, and then sit back and watch our muscles grow. This makes a good claim in an ad, but it doesn't translate into reality. Only through intense strength training can protein be utilized to repair and develop lean muscle tissue.

> *To effectively build muscle, we need to lift enough weight to challenge our muscles beyond their normal resistance levels.*

MYTH: High-protein diets are unnecessary for athletes.

WHY WE THINK THAT: Most athletes tend to engage in sports that require cardiovascular endurance, so we think of athletes as lean, sinewy figures who don't have a lot of muscle bulk. We also believe more protein equals bigger muscles.

THE FACTS: The United States Department of Agriculture (USDA) makes no distinction between the protein requirements of athletes, the average person, and complete couch potatoes. The RDA for protein is the same for all individuals, regardless of their activity levels.

However, studies have shown that athletes and people who exercise regularly do require a bit more protein than sedentary individuals. When we exercise, protein stores are broken down and used for fuel

> *Studies have shown that athletes and people who exercise regularly do require a bit more protein than sedentary individuals.*

through a process called gluconeogenesis. Research has shown that when athletes consume a low-protein diet, they do not have enough protein to repair and rebuild muscle tissue, thus their bodies will take the needed protein from other sources in the body, such as the organs. However, ingesting enormous quantities of protein will not improve athletic performance. A good formula for an athlete to follow for maximizing strength and performance is to consume approximately one gram of protein per day for each pound of body weight.

MYTH: Excess protein will be used as energy.

WHY WE THINK THAT: Again, we often believe what we

> *Consume approximately one gram of protein per day for each pound of body weight.*

hear or read without verifying the information. When we hear it or read it often enough, we believe it's the "truth."

THE FACTS: Protein is used by the body for energy only as a last resort, when carbohydrate and fat sources are depleted. Excess protein is stored as body fat.

MYTH: High-protein diets make you fat.

WHY WE THINK THAT: We often equate the word 'high" in reference to diet or food with "a lot." So, in our minds, a "high-protein diet" translates into "lots of protein in the diet." We all know that a lot of any food will make us fat.

THE FACTS: There is no doubt that eating too much protein will pack on the pounds, but so will eating too many calories from carbs or fat! If we consume more calories than we expend, we'll gain weight. Consequently, it's not more protein that causes weight gain it's the overconsumption of all calories. No matter what we eat, if we consume too much of it, we'll ultimately end up getting fat.

What to take away

- Protein is an essential nutrient used for building and repairing our bodies.
- We need complete proteins for our bodies to function properly.
- Excess protein will pack on the pounds, not muscle, if not used to maintain protein-containing tissues.
- Extra protein doesn't build more muscle. Muscle is built by activity, such as lifting more and heavier weights.

- Active people need only a little more protein than sedentary people.

9. FATS

American consumers have no problem with carcinogens, but they will not purchase any product, including floor wax, that has fat in it.

— Dave Barry

The only time to eat diet food is while you're waiting for the steak to cook.

— Julia Child

Fats and oils are part of a healthy diet, and should not be avoided. Most of us know that fats put taste, consistency, and stability into our foods and help us feel full. Our bodies need fats to function properly. Fats are used to produce and repair our cell membranes and the nervous system. Fats are needed to maintain healthy hair, nails, and skin. Fats also help to regulate blood pressure, heart rate, blood vessel constriction, and blood clotting. Without fats in our diet, we would not be able to extract vitamins A, D, E, and K from our foods.

The type of fat we consume does make a difference. Fats come in four basic types: monounsaturated, polyunsaturated, saturated, and trans fats. Polyunsaturated and monounsaturated fats, which are considered the healthiest, are found in fish, nuts, and plants. Saturated fats, such as butter, are solid at room temperature.

Fats and oils are part of a healthy diet, and should not be avoided.

Trans fats are monounsaturated or polyunsaturated oils that have either been chemically manipulated by the infusion of hydrogen, which makes them solid at room temperature or the result of superheating oils to make inexpensive, commercial oils with a long shelf life. Examples of hydrogenated trans fats are margarine and shortening used for baking. Trans fats are also found in many baked goods, such as crackers, potato chips, snack foods, boxed cereals, cake mixes, cookies, and pre-made dinners. Since trans fats contain nothing that will deteriorate, they are almost indestructible. Foods made with trans fats don't go rancid easily and can remain on store shelves, in our cabinets, and in our bodies for long periods of time. And no matter which way they were manufactured, trans fats are devoid of nutrients.

Since fats are used by our bodies to make and repair cells, it makes sense to consume them. Monounsaturated and polyunsaturated fats are important components of permeable cell membranes that allow nutrients to flow in and waste material to flow out of our cells. When saturated fats are used to make or repair cell membranes, the membrane becomes thicker and less permeable. Although this is useful for cells that facilitate clotting after an injury, it is not appropriate for all cells, thus it is recommended that our intake of saturated fats be limited. Trans fats can be used by our bodies to make and repair cells, but these cells are mutated and inferior. Mutated and inferior cells place a burden upon our immune system, and can form the beginnings of cancerous structures. Therefore, trans fats should be avoided.

> *Monounsaturated and polyunsaturated fats are important components of permeable cell membranes.*

Cholesterol is a soft, waxy kind of fat made by our bodies in the liver and is needed for normal body functions. It is the substance around which our steroid hormones, including estrogen and testosterone, are formed. It is essential for normal functioning of bile acids and vitamin D, which helps the body absorb bone-building calcium. Cholesterol is also required for cell building and is present in all parts of the body including the nervous system, skin, muscle, liver, intestines, and heart. The more physically active a person is, the more cholesterol the body will make. Cholesterol is a fat that uses two types of lipids to transport it in and out of a cell. The two types of transport lipids are HDL (high-density lipids) and LDL (low-density lipids). Think of HDLs as being a garbage truck that comes by the cell to take away waste products. HDL cholesterol acts like tiny little pellets that scrape the walls of our blood vessels, preventing plaque from building up. LDL cholesterol is like a UPS delivery truck that brings fat and energy to the cells. However, LDL is more like cotton candy. It's sticky and therefore attracts plaque, causing it to stick and build up on the inside walls of the blood vessels. HDL acts like an abrasive pad and scrubs the blood vessels clean as it moves through them. An ideal ratio is HDL/LDL above 0.4.

Triglycerides are another type of fat carried by the bloodstream. These are compounds used by the body to move fatty acids through

HDL acts like an abrasive pad and scrubs the blood vessels clean.

the blood. Fatty acids may be used by the body for energy or stored as fat for later use. Triglycerides are known to be bad for damaged arteries and are another component measured in a cholesterol or lipid test.

Even though cholesterol is a fat and HDL and LDL refer to how it is transported, for simplicity, I will refer to cholesterol in terms of how it is transported.

Fats that are naturally liquid at room temperature actually help our bodies to make good cholesterol (HDL) and decrease bad cholesterol (LDL). When saturated fats are consumed in large quantities for long periods of time, our bad cholesterol (LDL) may increase but our good cholesterol (HDL) will not decrease. Trans fats increase our bad cholesterol and lower our good cholesterol at the same time, even when consumed in small quantities.

Not only is the type of fat we ingest important, the amount we consume is also important. The typical Western or American diet is very high in fat, especially poor-quality saturated fats and trans fats.

The healthiest fats to consume are those found in walnut, peanut, olive, almond, grape seed, and sesame oils.

Remember that an excess of any macronutrient will be stored in the body as fat. For most people, total fat intake should be 20%-35% of the total diet. The typical, unhealthy, American diet contains 40% fat, much of which is trans fat.

But consuming too little fat creates problems, too. A diet containing less than 20% fat increases the risk of not getting enough of the essential fat-soluble vitamins A, D, E, and K. Decreasing our fat intake also leads to a reduced amount of good cholesterol (HDL) and elevates triglycerides. The healthiest fats to consume are those found in walnut, peanut, olive, almond, grape seed, and sesame oils. Other foods naturally high in healthy fats are nuts, olives, avocados, and certain types of fish.

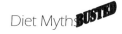

Table 5: Changing the plasma lipid profile.

You can raise HDL with
Alcohol, niacin, fibrates, statins, smoking cessation, estrogen, weight loss, and exercise.
The following will lower your HDL. Not something you want to do.
Certain drugs, smoking, progesterone, diabetes, obesity, metabolic syndrome, no exercise, high triglycerides.
You can lower your LDL with
Niacin, fibrates, statins, fat reduction, estrogen, weight loss, resins, bile acid sequestrants.
But avoid these things that will raise your LDL
Too many dietary fats, diabetes, obesity, thyroid disease, renal disease, liver disease. And be aware that genetics can be a factor.

Oils and fats are also referred to by type, such as omega-3, omega-6, and omega-9. These types of fats can help reduce the risk of heart disease. Omega-9 fats are found in monounsaturated oils, such as flax, olive, evening primrose, and borage oils. Not only do omega-9 fats reduce heart disease, they also help to reduce the risk of breast cancer, reduce LDL levels, and increase HDL levels. Omega-3 fats lower blood pressure and reduce the risk of heart attacks and strokes by making the blood less likely to form clots. Omega-3 fats also lower LDL and triglyceride levels while increasing HDL levels. Omega-3 fats are found in flaxseed, safflower, sunflower, corn, walnut, and other nut oils, and also in salmon, tuna, sardines, and many freshwater fish.

Omega-6 fats reduce the risk of heart disease by lowering LDL levels but can also lower HDL levels as well. Omega-6 fats are found in most vegetable oils, such as corn and soybean oils. The Western diet already contains more than enough omega-6, so it is best for all of us to get a better balance of all the omega types. Diets deficient in omega-3, -6, and -9 can result in flaky skin that itches, thin nails that split, dull hair, diarrhea, infections, inadequate growth, and slow healing.

> *Oils and fats are also referred to by type, such as omega-3, omega-6, and omega-9.*

In many diets, fats have received an undeserved reputation as villains because one gram of fat contains almost twice as many calories as one gram of carbohydrate or protein. Fats fill us up quickly and make us feel satisfied sooner than

> *In many diets, fats have received an undeserved reputation as villains.*

carbohydrates or proteins. When it comes to calories and added weight, excess calories of ANY macronutrient will pack on the pounds. Given the current obesity epidemic, it is clear that the low-fat diet has not worked due to excess consumption of all nutrients. All the macronutrients are important to our bodies, but they should be consumed in a balanced fashion and not eaten in excess.

Now for the myths.

MYTH: Consumption of fat is responsible for the obesity epidemic.

WHY WE THINK THAT: Since fat is a very calorie-dense nutrient, it would seem to make sense that consuming it would make us fat by doubling our calorie intake. Therefore, we think that eating fat always will make us fat.

THE FACTS: First, if this myth were true, with all the "low-fat" foods around, we should be getting slimmer instead of getting fatter, which is happening all over the world. Even though fat contains twice as many calories as carbohydrates per gram, the carbohydrates found in low-fat foods are stored as fat when overconsumed. When we eat too many carbohydrates, our blood sugar can rise to dangerously high levels. Insulin is produced to metabolize carbohydrates, first storing sugars as glycogen, then as fat. Insulin also blocks the release of the fat-burning hormone, glucagon. This metabolic roller coaster is directly responsible for the rise in diabetes, obesity, heart disease, cholesterol problems, chronic inflammation, and chronic fatigue syndrome that are now sweeping the globe.

MYTH: Fat should be eliminated from our diet.

WHY WE THINK THAT: Many fad diets emphasize the elimination of certain food groups perceived as having too much fat and advocate eating foods with as little fat as possible.

THE FACTS: Our bodies need a balanced diet that supplies us with diverse nutrients to keep us healthy. Our bodies need water, vitamins, protein, fat, minerals, carbohydrates, fiber, and oxygen. Eating a balanced diet that is rich in a variety of whole, unprocessed macronutrients will help us stay slimmer and healthier.

MYTH: All fats are bad for us.

WHY WE THINK THAT: For many decades we have been told by the American Heart Association that a diet containing fat gives us heart disease, so we should eliminate fat from our diets. When I was growing up, one of the heart surgeons my family knew wouldn't allow his family to eat beef, egg yolks, mayonnaise, butter, and other fats. Who's going to doubt a heart surgeon!?

THE FACTS: We all need fat because fats aid in nutrient absorption and nerve transmission, and help maintain cell membrane integrity and that's just a few of their useful purposes. Not all fats are created equal. Some fats can actually help promote good health, while others can increase our risk of heart disease. The key is to replace bad fats, such as poor-quality saturated fats, processed fats, and all trans fats, with good fats, such as natural saturated fats, monounsaturated fats, and polyunsaturated fats.

Some fats can actually help promote good health.

MYTH: Nuts are fattening.

WHY WE THINK THAT: They are! Nuts are high in calories. For instance, just fifteen cashews contain 180 calories and it is easy to eat too many!

THE FACTS: Nuts are high in monounsaturated and polyunsaturated fats, as well as plant sterols, all of which have been shown to lower LDL (bad) cholesterol levels. Nuts also contain healthy fats, such as omega-3, that raise our HDL (good cholesterol) levels and do not clog arteries. Nuts are good sources of protein, dietary fiber, and minerals, such as magnesium and copper. Though nuts are high in fat, they are very nutritious and are beneficial when consumed in moderation.

MYTH: Red meat contains bad types of fat and is bad for our health.

WHY WE THINK THAT: We have been told that red meat is linked with an increased risk of heart disease due to its saturated fat content.

FACTS: Moderate amounts of saturated fat from whole, unprocessed sources are not harmful. Saturated fat contains necessary vitamins used to rebuild cell structures and to promote blood-clotting abilities. If you are worried about your intake of saturated fat, it is important to understand that chicken can contain as much saturated fat as lean cuts of beef or pork. For example, a serving of beef sirloin or pork tenderloin has less saturated fat than the same size serving of a chicken thigh with skin. Poultry, such as chicken and turkey, is lower in saturated fat than red meat, but only if eaten without the skin. If you feel you need to reduce your intake of saturated fat, choose leaner cuts of beef, such as eye of round, top-round roast, top sirloin, tenderloin, or flank steak. For pork, choose tenderloin or loin chops.

Moderate amounts of saturated fat from whole, unprocessed sources are not harmful.

A rigorous experiment in Israel found that saturated fat isn't nearly as harmful as once thought. The people in the experiment were put on a low-carb, unrestricted-calorie diet, and consumed more saturated fat than a control group that cut back on both fat and calories. When the two groups were compared, the people who ate more saturated fat lost more weight and ended up with a better cholesterol profile.[14] This is just the latest in a series of studies contradicting the negative press about saturated fat.

MYTH: Fats and lean red meat cause cancer.

WHY WE THINK THAT: For decades the media and various medical groups have told us that red meat is bad for us, and we believe them because they are credible sources.

FACTS: Some studies of large populations have suggested a potential link between meat and cancer but, in reality, no study has ever found a direct cause-and-effect relationship between the consumption of red meat and cancer. The population studies are far from conclusive because they rely on broad surveys of people's eating habits and health afflictions, which are all different. Some people eat red meat with whole foods and also keep physically active, while others eat red meat with junk food and follow a sedentary lifestyle. The numbers are simply crunched to find trends, not causes. For example, in Argentina people have higher beef consumption than people in the United States, yet they have a lower rate of colon cancer. Mormons, who consume red meat, have lower rates of colon cancer than Seventh Day Adventists, who are vegetarians.

MYTH: Grilling meat causes cancer.

WHY WE THINK THAT: We believe rumors and what the media and research groups tell us.

THE FACTS: In 1986 Japanese researchers discovered cancer in rats that were fed heterocyclic amines (HCAs), which are compounds that are generated from overcooking red meat with high heat. HCAs mutate DNA and are suspected carcinogens.[15] The American Institute of Cancer Research (AICR) says that the risk of colorectal cancer increases 15% for every extra 1.7-ounce serving of grilled red meat.[16] However, using herbs from the Lamiaceae family, such as rosemary, sage, mint, basil, and oregano, may keep over-grilled meat from causing cancer. Researchers from Kansas State University found that meats that were marinated with rosemary before cooking contained 70-80% less HCAs than those not so marinated.[17]

When meat is overheated or grilled to the point of being burnt, unstable compounds called free radicals are produced from the meat's amino acids and sugars. The

Using herbs from the Lamiaceae family may keep over-grilled meat from causing cancer.

free radicals react with creatine (an organic acid created from amino acids and found in muscle) to make HCAs. The herbal antioxidants found in the Lamiaceae herbs stop the process. This may be why barbecue sauces are used when grilling meats. To stop HCAs from developing, coat the meat with barbeque sauce or marinate in spices before cooking.

You don't need to stop grilling meat, but treat it to an antioxidant bath before cooking, and don't burn it.

MYTH: Saturated fats clog arteries.

WHY WE THINK THAT: For decades the American Heart Association and the American Cancer Society have told us that saturated fats clog our arteries.

THE FACTS: In 1953 physiologist Dr. Ancel Keys proposed this hypothesis, but it has never been proven true. Keys was the inventor of the K-ration, the combat food of GIs during World War II. His hypothesis was based on observations of the dietary habits of businessmen in Minnesota and in 22 other countries. The data from only seven of the 23 countries supported his preconceived notion that saturated fat and cholesterol caused heart disease. Keys dismissed the data gathered from the other 16 countries because it contradicted his idea.[18] Ironically, before his death in 2004 he admitted that he skewed the results and acknowledged that dietary fat and cholesterol were unrelated to heart disease.

The fatty acids found in clogged arteries are mostly related to omega-6, which is found in processed vegetable oil and not in animal fat. Saturated fat makes up 54% of our cell membranes, giving them their shape, stiffness, and integrity.

> *Saturated fat makes up 54% of our cell membranes, giving them their shape, stiffness, and integrity.*

Saturated fatty acids enhance the immune system and help the body use omega-3. The fat around the heart muscle is saturated and is what the heart draws upon for energy when under stress.

MYTH: Saturated fat is the chief cause of heart disease.

WHY WE THINK THAT: We have been told by various well-established groups that saturated fat is the one main cause of coronary heart disease.

THE FACTS: Coronary heart disease (CHD) was not defined until 1910. Before that time, saturated fats were much more prevalent in our diets. At that time our saturated fats came from natural sources and we were much more physically active. People in northern India consume 17 times more animal fat than people in southern India, yet have 7 times less CHD.

East Africans drink ten liters of full-fat milk a day and have no CHD. Older Russian-Georgians consume the most saturated fat in the world and live to be very old. The people of Crete have a diet containing 40% saturated fat, yet have 95% fewer deaths from CHD than in the United States. The Masai tribes of Africa have no CHD, but their diet of meat, blood, and milk is high in saturated fat.

The Framingham Heart Study began in 1948, involved six thousand people, was run for forty years, and concluded: "We found that the people who ate the most saturated fat and cholesterol had the lowest levels of serum cholesterol, weighed the least, and were the most active."

A recent study, done through the collaboration of numerous research facilities at many universities, investigated the effects of dietary fats and carbohydrates on the development of coronary atherosclerosis in postmenopausal women. Those who consumed a higher carbohydrate diet had a greater risk of developing heart disease than those who ate a diet with higher concentrations of saturated fat.[19]

> *Those who consumed a higher carbohydrate diet had a greater risk of developing heart disease than those who ate a diet with higher concentrations of saturated fat.*

MYTH: Since other societies have adopted our Western diet, their people's risks for heart disease, cancer, obesity, and diabetes have also increased.

WHY WE THINK THAT: Pictures don't lie. We see more and more overweight people in countries and cultures that didn't seem to have that problem before.

THE FACTS: It is true that, as other societies adopt our Western diet, their people become overweight and obese. Unfortunately, they also adopt our Western lifestyle. That means eating more refined foods, eating more sugar, eating too much too often, eating too many calories, and being a lot less active.

MYTH: Coconut oil causes heart disease.

WHY WE THINK THAT: Since coconut oil is a saturated fat and we tend to believe that saturated fat causes heart disease, we logically think that coconut oil causes heart disease. One myth feeds into another.

THE FACTS: When patients recovering from heart attacks were fed a diet containing 7% coconut oil, they had greater improvement compared to untreated controls, and there was no difference between those fed coconut oil and patients fed corn oil or safflower oil.[20] Populations that consume coconut oil as a regular part of their diets have lower rates of heart disease. Coconut oil helps to prevent heart disease because it has antiviral and antimicrobial characteristics.

> *Populations that consume coconut oil as a regular part of their diets have lower rates of heart disease.*

MYTH: Saturated fats inhibit the production of prostaglandins that inhibit inflammation.

WHY WE THINK THAT: Heart disease, some cancers, diabetes, and arthritis are caused by inflammatory conditions. For example, heart disease is caused by arteries that are narrowed by swollen, inflamed walls. To prevent these diseases, we need a diet that encourages our bodies to resist inflammation. Since saturated fats appear dense and hard, we assume they cause inflammation.

THE FACTS: Saturated fats facilitate the production of essential fatty acids, which go on to improve the production of prostaglandins. Prostaglandins are hormone-like fatty compounds in our bodies that help to control blood pressure, inflammation, and muscle movement. Arachidonic acid, an essential, unsaturated fatty acid that is necessary for the production of prostaglandins, is found in foods such as meat, liver, butter, and egg yolks.

MYTH: Foods that contain "zero trans fat" contain good fats.

WHY WE THINK THAT: We like to think we can believe what we read. We assume that if there is no trans fat in a food, the remaining fats are good.

THE FACTS: Don't assume that a "trans-fat free" food is a healthy choice. By law, a product can contain up to one-half gram of trans fat per serving and still say it has "zero" trans fat. If we eat a larger portion, we might be getting more trans fat than we think.

MYTH: Olive oil has fewer calories than other fats.

WHY WE THINK THAT: Since olive oil is healthy oil, we would like to believe it has fewer calories.

THE FACTS: All oils are 100% fat and supply the same number of calories, specifically 120 calories per tablespoon. "Light" olive oil

> *All oils are 100% fat and supply the same number of calories.*

does not have fewer calories than regular olive oil; "light" simply refers to the flavor, which is not as strong as that of regular olive oil. Even though olive oil is a good source of monounsaturated fats, it is still a fat and should be used in moderation.

MYTH: Low-fat or nonfat means no calories.

WHY WE THINK THAT: We tend to assume that "low-fat" and "nonfat" mean that food won't make us fat.

THE FACTS: A low-fat or nonfat food is not necessarily lower in calories than the same-sized portion of the full-fat product. When fat is taken out, something else is usually put back in. Many low fat or nonfat foods contain added sugar, flour, or starch to improve the flavor and texture after the fat is removed. These ingredients add calories but lack nutrition. Some studies suggest that snacks with low-fat labels entice us to indulge in more helpings or larger servings. We end up eating more food, and thus more calories, than if we selected the regular, full-fat version. Plus, low fat and nonfat foods don't satisfy us, as they don't give us that full, satiated feeling, so we eat more.

MYTH: Low-fat diets prevent breast cancer.

WHY WE THINK THAT: We believe that fat is the enemy food and is the root cause of many of our diseases.

THE FACTS: A recent study found that women on diets with less than 20% fat had the same rate of

> *Low-fat diets don't affect our risk for getting breast cancer.*

breast cancer as women who consumed a diet with larger amounts of fat. Low-fat diets don't affect our risk for getting breast cancer.

MYTH: Low-fat diets make us feel better.

WHY WE THINK THAT: Many of us think fat is the cause of all of our nutritional problems, including why we are overweight.

THE FACTS: Recent studies showed that a high intake of refined starches and sugars found in low-fat foods increases a person's risk for diabetes, heart disease, and obesity. People who are obese run a higher risk of throat cancer; refined carbohydrates are thought to be the cause. Research shows that cancer cells prefer sugar as a fuel, over proteins and fats.

On a more positive note, our body performs better and we feel better when quality fats make up around 25-30% of our total calories and when our carbohydrates come from whole, unrefined sources.

MYTH: To prevent heart disease, eat margarine instead of butter.

WHY WE THINK THAT: Since butter is a saturated fat, and we believe saturated fat is one main cause of heart disease, we tend to choose margarine over butter.

THE FACTS: People who eat margarine have twice the rate of heart disease compared to people who eat butter. Margarine and butter contain different types of fat. Margarine is lower in saturated fat than butter, but contains hydrogenated fats. Hydrogenated fats are much more harmful to our health than whole, natural sources of saturated fats, such as butter.

People who eat margarine have twice the rate of heart disease compared to people who eat butter.

MYTH: Eating a high-fat diet and/or excessive amounts of chocolate will cause acne.

WHY WE THINK THAT: People with acne often have oily skin and clogged pores. Fat is also oily, so we assume eating oily or greasy food causes our skin to become oily. In its sweetened form, chocolate is high in calories and fat, so we equate the fat with oil production of the skin.

Chocolate is an antioxidant, and the darker it is, the better.

THE FACTS: This has never been proven to be true. Acne is caused by a combination of bacteria, hormones, and family history. Chocolate is an antioxidant, and the darker it is, the better. Chocolate is not so bad; the processed sugar and fats added to the chocolate make it into a junk food and cause an imbalance in our hormones. Excessive amounts of sugar, especially high-fructose corn syrup (HFCS), have been shown to cause our skin to lose its flexibility and its firming tissue, collagen, as well as causing hormonal imbalances. Cocoa is the pure, unprocessed form of chocolate. The Mayans used cocoa to tenderize meat and made it into a strong tea with hot, red peppers. The Europeans imported cocoa and added sugar, cream, and fat to make it the sweet treat it has become.

MYTH: Low-fat foods are healthier for us.

WHY WE BELIEVE THAT: This propaganda has many people confused about their food choices. We buy processed, hybridized, modified, low-fat foods and then microwave them. Such food is so unnatural that we might as well eat cardboard.

THE FACTS: Fat is necessary for the uptake of many nutrients, particularly the fat-soluble vitamins A, E, D, and K, and the numerous

Without fat we cannot produce certain hormones.

carotenoids. Without fat we cannot produce certain hormones. Symptoms of hormone imbalance have been on the rise over the past 30-40 years.

What to take away

- Fats are essential to our diet and, in themselves, will not make us fat. Excess calories will make us fat.
- The best fat choices for maintaining our bodily systems are natural monounsaturated and polyunsaturated fats.
- Like any other macronutrient, when fats are consumed in excessive amounts, they contribute to weight gain.
- Saturated fats are not the root cause of heart disease and cancer; trans fats are far more likely to cause these ailments. Trans fats, whether hydrogenated or superheated oils, should be avoided.

10. WATER

Water, taken in moderation, cannot hurt anybody.
— Mark Twain

Ever wonder about those people who spend $2 apiece on those little bottles of Evian water? Try spelling Evian backward.
— George Carlin

In the United States we have the cleanest, best drinking water in the world and it comes from our faucets and drinking fountains. Yet Americans spend more than $15 billion a year on bottled water, thinking it is healthier. Let's look at some of the myths about water so you can make more informed decisions.

MYTH: Bottled water is better than tap water.

WHY WE BELIEVE THAT: Bottled water comes in fancy containers with pictures of pristine scenery on the labels and offers promises of purity and health, so we think it must be better. Why would smart people like us pay for anything less?

THE FACTS: Bottled water is not necessarily better. While advertisers brag about how bottled water starts as a snowflake or flows from *Bottled water is not necessarily better.* pure mountain streams, in reality all water is recycled from rain or snow, and has been for billions of years. Yep, we are drinking very old water. Twenty-five percent to forty percent of bottled water comes from less exotic-sounding sources. Bottled water generally comes from U.S. municipal water supplies. Bottling companies buy the water, filter it, and some add minerals. It's not really a bad thing since the Environmental Protection Agency (EPA) oversees municipal water quality and the Food and Drug Administration (FDA) monitors bottled water. In some cases EPA codes are more stringent, so bottled water's marketing borders on false advertising since bottling companies brag about their sources

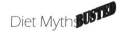

(which may or may not be exactly the same as the sources we have). If they can get water from the tap, so can we.

MYTH: Purified water tastes better.

WHY WE THINK THAT: When it comes to water or anything we drink, we associate "purified" with "clean." We all want to drink clean water.

THE FACTS: The "purest" water is distilled water; since all the minerals and salts have been removed, it tastes flat. It's the sodium, calcium, magnesium, and chloride that give water its flavor. Hard water often has an "iron" taste to it. The "off" taste of tap water is from the chlorine. If you refrigerate tap water in a container with a loose-fitting lid, the chlorine taste will be gone overnight. Since taste is subjective, taste is up to the individual.

> *It's the sodium, calcium, magnesium, and chloride that give water its flavor.*

MYTH: Bottled water with vitamins, minerals, or protein is healthier than regular water.

WHY WE THINK THAT: We believe we are getting more of what we think we need in just one drink of water and, since water has no calories, we are getting positive nutrition without getting more calories.

THE FACTS: "Vitamins, color, herbs, protein, and all the other additions to water, those are a marketing ploy," says Marion Nestle, PhD, professor of nutrition studies at New York University. The additives provide only a scant serving of the vitamins we need in a day and therefore make no nutritional impact. Enhanced waters may contain sugars and artificial flavorings to enhance their taste, and some have more calories than diet soda, but, because it is water, we ignore the calories. When it comes to providing fluoride, tap water usually wins, though that element is increasingly being added to bottled waters. Go ahead and drink bottled water, just read the label carefully.

MYTH: You need eight eight-ounce glasses of water each day.

WHY WE THINK THAT: For decades the media and trusted professionals in the medical and fitness fields have told us that we should drink at least eight 8-ounce glasses of water per day. As a fitness professional, I told my classes this and followed this advice myself for a long time.

THE FACTS: The Institute of Medicine recommends a total of about 91 ounces, or a little more than eleven 8-ounce glasses, of fluid daily for women. The liquid can come from water, juice, coffee, tea, or other beverages, along with liquids contained in solid foods. You need to replace the water you excrete through sweat, elimination, and breathing, but that doesn't add up to as much as 64 ounces of water. This myth came about because a 1947 study showed that the average intake from food for the average person is around 2,000 calories, and it takes about 64 ounces of liquid to process that. However, much of the necessary liquid is found in the food itself in the form of water in fruits, vegetables, meats, and cheeses.[21]

Is there scientific evidence for "8 x 8"? It is not necessary to drink an additional 64 ounces. However, the more active you are, the thirstier you may get, so drinking water is beneficial. A good rule to follow is if your urine is pale yellow, you are hydrated. If it is darker, drink more water.

MYTH: After an intense workout, bottled water is best.

WHY WE THINK THAT: See the previous myth about minerals, vitamins, and nutrients added to bottled water. We are all susceptible to what advertisers want us to think about their products.

THE FACTS: There's a reason volunteers hand out Gatorade during marathons. If our workout is intense and lasts longer than an hour, we need to replace the water and elec-

If our workout is intense and lasts longer than an hour, we need to replace water and electrolytes.

trolytes, such as sodium and potassium, which we've lost. We can do that with solid food or with liquids such as 100% fruit juice or fortified drinks. For less intense workouts, regular tap water is fine.

MYTH: Drinking lots of water helps the kidneys clear out toxins.

WHY WE THINK THAT: Since kidneys are our filtering system, we think if we flush our system with water like we flush our toilets and septic systems, we are helping our own systems.

THE FACTS: The kidneys filter toxins from our bloodstreams. Then the toxins are cleared out through the urine. The body can use only a certain amount of liquid or water at any given time. Drinking too much water reduces the kidney's ability to function as a filter and can eventually cause the brain to swell, stopping it from regulating vital functions such as breathing, and eventually causing death. After water enters the body, it is removed primarily in the urine and sweat. The amount of water in the body is regulated by the body to control the levels of certain compounds, such as salt, in the blood.

If we drink too much water, the kidneys eventually will not be able to work fast enough to remove sufficient amounts of water from the body, so the levels of salt and other chemicals in the blood become diluted.

> After water enters the body, it is removed primarily in the urine and sweat.

This leads to swelling of the organs including the brain. The brain is then pushed up against the walls of the skull. The resulting increase in pressure causes a loss of brain function to the point that vital functions, such as breathing, cease. (It takes a lot of water to do that. As Mark Twain said, be sure to drink water in moderation.)

MYTH: Drinking lots of water will gives us healthier skin.

WHY WE THINK THAT: We believe if we drink those eight glasses of water a day, we will improve our health, and that will show in our skin.

THE FACTS: The body is already 70-75% water. So, if you take a 200-pound man, he's 150 pounds of water. Adding a few extra glasses of water each day has a limited effect. "Although frank dehydration can obviously decrease skin turgor, or the ability for skin to bounce back, it is not clear what benefit drinking extra water has for skin," say Dan Negoianu and Stanley Goldfarb in their editorial in the June 2008 issue of the *Journal of the American Society of Nephrology*.[22] "One study suggested ingestion of 500 ml of water increases…capillary blood flow in the skin. It is unclear whether these changes are clinically significant…We were unable to find any other data regarding the impact of water intake on skin in otherwise healthy people."

MYTH: Drinking extra water leads to weight loss.

WHY WE THINK THAT: We have read that drinking water breaks down our fat stores and helps us metabolize our food better.

THE FACTS: A more accurate statement is that drinking water may be a helpful tool for dieters. "Water is a great strategy for dieters because it has no calories," says Madeline Fernstrom of the University of Pittsburgh.[23] "So you can keep your mouth busy without food and get the sense of satisfaction. But water is not magical." Water will give us a feeling of being full for a short amount of time, but it might be enough time to let us wait a little longer before we eat again. However, if we think it is a "magic bullet," we run the risk of using it as an excuse for not making needed changes in our eating behaviors and we may drink too much.

MYTH: It's easy to get dehydrated during a workout.

WHY WE THINK THAT: Look around any fitness club or gym and we'll see vending machines selling bottled water, so we are led to believe we need a constant supply of water all the time.

THE FACTS: Dehydration sets in when a person has lost 2% of his or her body weight by sweating. So for a 200-pound man, this means losing four pounds of water.

> Marathon runners, bikers, and hikers all need to recognize the signs of dehydration.

Marathon runners, bikers, and hikers all need to recognize the signs of dehydration. Individuals in hot, dry climates have an increased need for water. The American College of Sports Medicine recommends that athletes drink sixteen ounces of fluids a couple of hours before starting sports practice.[24]

For a stroll in the park or a trip to the mall, no water bottle is necessary. The best advice: drink when you're thirsty.

MYTH: All bottled water, whether tonic, sparkling, flavored, or mineral, is the same as plain water.

WHY WE THINK THAT: Since water contains no calories, and flavored water is still water, we are able to delude ourselves that it is all the same as far as calories are concerned.

THE FACTS: Plain bottled water is calorie-free and also fluoride-free, so be sure to get fluoride from other sources. Tonic water, which contains quinine and sugar, has 125 calories per serving. Flavored waters contain sugar and fruit juice, and therefore calories, so read the label. Some flavored waters are made with artificial sweeteners and flavors; while they don't contain calories, they are not necessarily healthy.

MYTH: Diet water is real.

WHY WE THINK THAT: We are all looking for a "magic pill" or "magic drink" that will let us avoid the real work of keeping ourselves fit and at a proper weight through diet and exercise. Isn't it interesting that every time a new weight-loss product is introduced, it is either a food or a drink to be consumed, when the problem is overconsumption itself?

THE FACTS: Americans bought and consumed 26 billion liters of water in 2004, and the number has been steadily increasing since. At the moment there are 150

When the water is consumed thirty minutes before eating, a person will feel less hungry and consume less.

different brands of bottled waters on the market, and the companies that produce them keep coming up with new methods of making themselves competitive with each other. One of the newest concepts in the business of selling "healthy" water is Jana's Skinny Water. Jana claims that their Skinny Water contains an ingredient from an artesian well in Croatia that makes the body burn more calories after the water is consumed. The only real claim that Jana can make is that when the water is consumed thirty minutes before eating, a person will feel less hungry and consume less. However, that same claim is valid whether a person drinks bottled water or tap water. The *Journal of the American Medical Association* published a study that compared the weight loss of people who drank Skinny Water with tap water and concluded there was no significant difference.[25]

Other manufacturers of diet water add stimulants to suppress the appetite. However, once the stimulant wears off, the consumer is left with a big appetite and is likely to overeat to compensate. Stimulants can disrupt one's sleeping patterns, and disrupted sleep causes the appetite to increase. Just use common sense: how can something that is already calorie-free be less so?

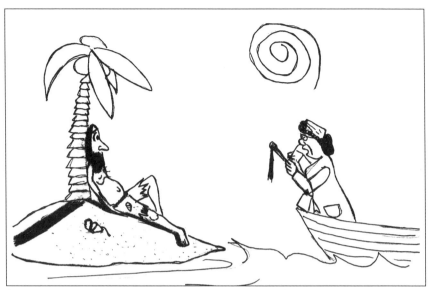

So, do you prefer tap water, bottled water, or flavored water?

"Healthy" water to avoid: Glaceau Vitamin Water (any flavor; 20-ounce bottle), 130 calories, 33 grams of sugar. Vitamins and water might sound like the ultimate nutritional-dream team, but a bottle of this water carries as much sugar and calories as a can of soda pop. Makes sense, though, since this so-called functional beverage is produced by the Coca-Cola Company. You should avoid other sugary healthy water, too.

What to take away

- Most bottled water is tap water, so buy it for convenience, not health.
- Enhanced water doesn't have enough nutrition to matter.
- There is no such thing as "diet water" that really works.

11. SODA POP

> More people die in the United States of too much food than of too little.
>
> — John Kenneth Galbraith

As a nation we spent $68.1 billion on soda pop in 2009. According to the Beverage Marketing Association, every man, woman, and child in the United States ingests 192 gallons of liquid a year. That translates into about 3.7 gallons per week or just over two quarts per day. Of those two quarts, 28% of the liquid consumed is from carbonated soft drinks. To visualize this amount of pop consumed per year, think of a standard-size bathtub that holds 30-32 gallons of water. All of this pop is nothing but water plus refined, nutrient-deficient sugar. Now imagine the effect of three tubs full of soft drink on the teeth and the body. Over one fourth of our yearly liquid intake is of questionable nutritional value, and contributes to a variety of health issues, including diabetes, obesity, cavities, tooth decay, and osteoporosis.

Fifty years ago the average serving of soda pop was 6.5 ounces and it was considered a treat. Ten years later, the standard size for *Fifty years ago the average serving of soda pop was 6.5 ounces.* soda pop had almost doubled, in the form of 12-ounce cans. Today, soft drinks are a regular part of our daily dietary intake, with the average serving size being 20-24 ounces and many servings exceed 36 ounces. At the movies, we can get a 44-ounce serving of soda. That is the same size as the Super Big Gulp offered by 7-Eleven, which costs only 25 cents more than a 32-ounce "medium," making it an "exceptional" value.

Along with the increase in serving size, the consumption rate of soda pop has increased dramatically among teenagers and young adult consumers. Thirty years ago teenage boys consumed twice as much milk as sodas and teenage girls consumed one-and-a-half times more milk than other beverages. Today, teenagers drink twice as much soda pop as milk.

Soda pop has replaced nutrient-dense beverages and water as a preferred drink and, since sodas don't contain vitamins, minerals, or dietary fiber, researchers believe this dietary shift is a major factor in the rising numbers of overweight and obese teens. Currently at least 65% of all teens are either overweight or obese. As a result of this increase in obesity, type II diabetes has skyrocketed among teens and the young adult population, especially among females. Excess weight gain has a significant impact on cardiovascular health and cancer rates. Obese teens are now suffering from fatty liver disease, a condition once seen only in sedentary adults.

Frequent consumption of soda pop may lead to an increased incidence of bone fractures among young adults or the development of osteoporosis in later life, since the decreased consumption of milk reduces calcium intake. Bone mass is built in early life, and women reach more than 90% of their bone density by their late teens. With the decreased consumption of milk and the increased intake of soft drinks over the last three decades, calcium intake among today's teenage girls and young-adult women is well below recommended rates, creating risk for a definite increase in bone fractures.

Women reach more than 90% of their bone density by their late teens.

I received proof of that when we went to South Carolina to attend our daughter's graduation from Army Basic Combat Training at Fort Jackson. Our daughter was amazed at how many of the young men and women suffered stress fractures and bone fractures incurred after executing basic exercises. When she inquired about their dietary habits, she found out that many of them drank soda pop as their main choice of beverage instead of water or milk. Most almost never drank milk.

Soda pop is a staple of a high-sugar diet. When adults consume a diet high in sugars and triglycerides, insulin levels rise. High-sugar diets cause inflammation of the arteries, which causes a narrowing of the passageways, thus contributing to heart disease. Studies associate high levels of triglycerides with an increased risk for cardiovascular disease and diabetes.

Researchers have looked at the role of coffee, tea, and soda pop in the formation of kidney stones, a painful disorder that affects 10% of all

Americans some time in their lives. Young men, the heaviest consumers of soft drinks, are much more likely to suffer from this painful disorder than women. Manufacturers add caffeine, a mild stimulant, to the majority of sodas, claiming that caffeine adds flavor. Caffeine has no flavor activity in soft drinks, yet will induce a physiological and psychological desire to consume the drink. Consuming two to three cans of soda pop results in the ingestion of 100 milligrams of caffeine per day, which is not good for anyone suffering from kidney stones. New soft-drink products are being introduced that contain two to three times the level of caffeine found in traditional soda pop. Since caffeine is mildly addictive, people who drink lots of soda may also be addicted.

Artificial colors, sweeteners, and preservatives are suspected of causing allergic reactions, aggravating attention-deficit hyperactivity disorder (ADHD) in sensitive individuals, and producing carcinogenic compounds. Dental professionals are particularly concerned about the acid (pH) levels and sugar content of soft drinks. Carbonated and noncarbonated soft drinks, as well as those that contain sugar and those classified as sugar-free, contain various amounts of phosphoric, citric, and carbonic acids, and can be responsible for significant tooth demineralization. A 12-ounce serving of soda pop contains 9.6-11 teaspoons of sugar, which is fermented by oral bacteria, thus increasing the amount of acid in our mouths.

Manufacturers of soft drinks spend millions of dollars every year marketing their products through print, television, billboards, and radio. Soft drinks of all types are readily available from vending machines, fast-food restaurants, convenience stores, and through school-based programs. Grocery stores run weekly specials on soft drinks, an already inexpensive beverage. This means cash-strapped families can purchase a two-liter (2.1-quart) bottle of soda for 59 cents, or get it free with a coupon, when a half-gallon of milk may cost $2.19.

Manufacturers of soft drinks spend millions of dollars every year marketing their products.

Although sales of high-sugar soft drinks have slipped in favor of diet sodas and bottled water, soda manufacturers are adding trace amounts of nutrients to their carbonated beverages in an effort to appear "healthy."

New products include beverages with large amounts of caffeine and ginseng additives. So-called "fortified beverages" contain trace amounts of vitamins B_3, B_6, B_{12}, and E, and metals, such as chromium, magnesium, and zinc. These additives are not present in any amounts that matter and do not offset the effects of the abundance of sugar in the soda.

Diet pop and artificial sweeteners don't give us much help with losing weight and becoming healthy. Dr. Susan Swithers and Dr. Terry Davidson, psychologists at

Diet pop and artificial sweeteners don't give us much help with losing weight and becoming healthy.

Purdue University's Ingestive Behavior Research Center, reported that compared to rats given fully sweetened yogurt, rats given yogurt sweetened with zero-calorie saccharin later consumed significantly more calories, gained more weight, put on more body fat, and didn't make up for it by cutting back later.

Swithers and Davidson surmised that by breaking the connection between a sweet sensation and high-calorie food, the use of artificial sweeteners changes the body's ability to regulate intake. Three different experiments explored whether artificial sweeteners changed lab animals' ability to regulate their intake, using different assessments, the most obvious being caloric intake, weight gain, and compensating by cutting back. The experimenters also measured changes in core body temperature, a physiological assessment. Normally when we prepare to eat, our metabolic engine revs up, thus creating heat. However, rats that had been trained to respond to saccharin, compared to rats trained to respond to sugar, showed a smaller rise in core body temperate after eating a novel, sweet-tasting, high-calorie meal. The authors think this blunted response led to overeating and also made it harder to burn off sweet-tasting calories.

"The data clearly indicate that consuming a food sweetened with no-calorie saccharin can lead to greater body-weight gain and adiposity than would consuming the same food sweetened with a higher-calorie sugar." Swithers and Davidson also wrote that "other artificial sweeteners such as aspartame, sucralose, and acesulfame K, which also taste sweet but do not predict the delivery of calories, could have similar effects." The findings match emerging evidence that people who consume diet drinks

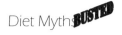

in an effort to lose weight are at higher risk for obesity and metabolic syndrome. Metabolic syndrome is characterized by increased abdominal fat, high blood pressure, and insulin resistance, all of which put people at risk for heart disease and diabetes.

Why would a sugar substitute backfire? Swithers and Davidson wrote that sweet foods provide a "salient orosensory stimulus" that strongly predicts someone is about

People who consume diet drinks in an effort to lose weight are at higher risk for obesity.

to take in a lot of calories. Ingestive and digestive reflexes prepare for a sweet intake and the calories that come with it, but when sweetness is not accompanied by calories, the system gets confused. Thus, people may eat more or expend less energy than they otherwise would.

The good news, Swithers says, is that people can still count calories to regulate intake and body weight. However, she sympathizes with the dieter's lament that counting calories requires more conscious effort than consuming low-calorie foods. So, the lesson is "buyer beware" when selecting beverages.

The desire for a sweet drink is natural. "We are born with a taste for sweet because breast milk is sweet," explains Samantha Heller, senior clinical nutritionist at New York University Medical Center.[26] "When we start feeding sweets and soda to infants and toddlers, we're taking the natural instinct for a sweet taste and intensifying that desire. Soon, even the sweet taste of fruit is not enough for the children; they want extreme sweets, like soda." The effect of training our bodies to crave sugary soda and other sweetened foods lasts long past childhood.

Nobody is saying that soft drinks are solely to blame for America's obesity problem, but a new study confirms that they are a key part. In the two decades from 1977 to 1997, childhood obesity rates doubled. At the same time, the amount of soda pop consumed by kids also doubled. That's not a coincidence. A report published in the *American Journal of Clinical Nutrition* analyzed thirty studies on nutrition over the past forty years and found strong evidence that soda is making Americans fat. That extra weight puts Americans at risk for heart disease, diabetes, stroke, and cancer and helps to send health care costs through the roof.

Children are especially vulnerable because they don't fully comprehend the hazards of consuming too much sugary soda. But children are not the only ones affected; adults are affected, too.

Soda is making Americans fat.

The primary fault does not lie with soda-makers; it lies with those who choose to consume too many fattening soft drinks. The solution is simple: we must make better choices. The information we need is right on the can.

Now for the myths:

MYTH: Diet pop is healthier than regular pop.

WHY WE THINK THAT: Regular pop has more calories than diet pop and we know that less weight means being healthier, so we think diet pop will help us keep our weight down.

THE FACTS: A can of regular pop has 135 calories and a diet pop has 10 calories or even no calories. So regular pop contains more calories than diet pop, but diet pop contains artificial sweeteners and colors that

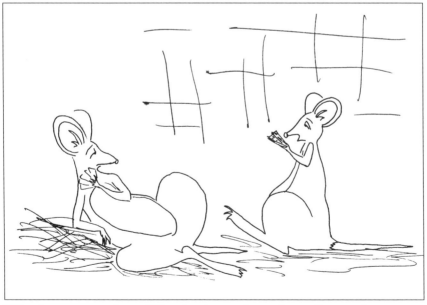

I'll raise you one dose of Saccharine and one dose of sugar to your Aspartame.

are not healthy. Aspartame has been associated with a higher risk of having babies with phenylketonuria (PKU).

According to a recent study, diet pop is linked to all the same health problems as regular pop. Research-

> *Diet pop is linked to all the same health problems as regular pop.*

ers from Boston University studied data from more than 6,000 middle-aged adults participating in the large-scale Framingham Heart Study.[27] These participants were all free of metabolic syndrome at the start of the study. Metabolic syndrome is a cluster of symptoms, such as excessive fat around the waist, impaired fasting glucose, high blood pressure, low levels of "good" HDL cholesterol. After four years of follow up, researchers found that adults who drank one or more sodas a day, regardless if the soda was diet or regular, had about a 50% higher risk of metabolic syndrome.

Prior studies linked consumption of regular pop and its high levels of sugar with multiple risk factors for heart disease. Soda is sweetened with high-fructose corn syrup. HFCS is an easy and cheap sweetener to manufacture, and it's been linked to obesity. The consumption of HFCS and the obesity rate have risen in parallel.

Diet pop is not a healthy alternative. The Framingham study was the first to find that the link to heart disease extends to low-calorie diet pop. The most intriguing fact researchers found was that participants who drink one or more sodas a day, again regular or diet, had a 31% greater risk of becoming overweight.

Diet soft drinks are not the panacea they appear to be. Researchers found evidence that the widespread use of no-calorie sweeteners may actually make it harder for people to control their calorie intake and, therefore, their body weight. The artificial sweeteners break the link between the taste for sweetness and calorie intake. With no signal to stop, a person eats too much. Here are the basic ingredients found in most diet sodas:

- Calories: 0
- Caffeine: varies from 0 to 55 mg. per can
- Carbonated Water
- Caramel color

- Sodium Benzoate
- Artificial Sweeteners (Aspartame or Acesulfame Potassium)
- Natural Flavor
- Artificial Flavor
- Sodium Citrate
- Malic Acid

MYTH: Regular pop is better than diet pop.
WHY WE THINK THAT: Even though diet pop has little or no calories, it is sweetened with chemicals, which we believe are unhealthy.

THE FACTS: Both diet and regular pop outrank coffee as America's favorite beverages. Neither is healthy, as they both increase the risks of kidney and heart disease, plus they contain acids that erode

> *By substituting a bottle of water instead of a can of pop or a can of juice, we can lose as many as 15 pounds per year.*

tooth enamel, thus causing tooth decay. By substituting a bottle of water instead of a can of pop or a can of juice, we can lose as many as 15 pounds per year. When purchasing a bottled or canned drink, be sure to read the label. Try to drink water instead of choosing a drink from a vending machine. This will save on your wallet and your waistline. Here are the basic ingredients found in a regular 12 oz. can of soda pop:

- 150 empty calories
- carbonated water
- fructose
- caffeine
- sugar
- flavoring
- phosphoric acid

MYTH: Soda pop weakens the bones.
WHY WE THINK THAT: Recent articles in popular magazines have warned us against drinking soda pop because the carbonization leaches calcium from our bones or prevents us from absorbing calcium from our foods.

THE FACTS: This "myth" is absolutely true. A study reported in 2006 by researchers at Tufts University in Boston suggests that dark colas are a problem.[28] Among the

> *Drinking soda pop leaches calcium from our bones.*

1,413 women whose dietary records and bone-density scans were reviewed, those who drank a diet or regular cola at least three times a week over five years had significantly lower bone densities than those who sipped cola once a month or less. No such effect occurred with other carbonated drinks, even after researchers factored in intake of calcium from foods.

The culprit is phosphoric acid, according to Katherine Tucker, PhD, lead author of the study. Although found in all carbonated drinks, phosphoric acid is more abundant in dark colas. When the body breaks down this compound, the acidity of the blood increases. To neutralize acidity, hydrogen ions bind with minerals, including calcium and magnesium. If these minerals are not available in the blood, Tucker says, "The body draws calcium from bones." The occasional cola drinker probably needn't worry. "The real risk is for those who drink cola every day," says Tucker.

MYTH: Drinking fruit juice is better than drinking soda pop.

WHY WE THINK THAT: Since soda is just sugar water, juice is better since its sugars come from fruits, which have nutrients and vitamins.

THE FACTS: Fruit juice, either fresh-squeezed or from 100% pure sources, is more nutritious, but it is still pure sugar to our body, just like soda pop. Like soda, juice is easy to overconsume and will cause cavities in teeth, just like soda pop. Many juices look healthy but are really just a fruit-flavored mixture of sugar and water containing very little real fruit juice and are chemically fortified with vitamins and nutrients.

Juice imposter to avoid: Arizona Kiwi Strawberry (23.5-ounce can), 360 calories, 84 grams of sugar. All of these fruit juice imposters should be avoided. Many contain only 5% juice and are 95% sugar water. They are sold at gas stations and convenience stores all across America for less than a dollar, making them among the cheapest sources of empty calories in the country.

Smoothie to avoid: Jamba Juice Peanut Butter Moo'd Power Smoothie (30 ounces), 1,170 calories, 69 grams of sugars, 30 grams of fat. Jamba Juice calls it a smoothie; but I call it a milkshake. It has more sugar than an entire bag of chocolate chips, and doesn't contain ANY juice. Watch out for similar products in other disguises.

What to take away

- Whether diet or regular, soda pop is not a healthy beverage choice and is a prime source of empty calories.
- Whether diet or regular, pop contributes to weight gain.
- Fruit juice is not always a healthy alternative and contains lots of unnecessary calories.

12. Coffee, Tea, And Caffeine

I never drink coffee at lunch. I find it keeps me awake for the afternoon.

— Ronald Reagan

Woman seated next to Winston Churchill: "If you were my husband, I'd poison your tea!"
Mr. Churchill: "And if you were my wife, I would drink it!"

Coffee, once thought to be a health pariah, has been the subject of more than 19,000 studies during the past 50 years. Rather than prove coffee to be unhealthy, the research has uncovered a number of healthful benefits for regular coffee drinkers. Here are the health benefits of coffee:

- Long-term consumption reduces the risk of type II diabetes.
- Protects premenopausal women against breast cancer.
- Reduces the risk of colon, liver, and bladder cancer.
- Inhibits inflammation in postmenopausal women, thereby helping to prevent cardiovascular disease.
- May protect against Alzheimer's disease.
- Lowers the risk of Parkinson's disease.
- Does not increase the risk of coronary heart disease.
- May help prevent gallstones.

> *Research has uncovered a number of healthful benefits for regular coffee drinkers.*

Let's get right to the myths about coffee, tea, and caffeine:

MYTH: Coffee contains little or no nutritional value.
WHY WE THINK THAT: With all the different studies that have been put out over the decades, it is hard to know what to think about

coffee, but since it has no calories, it would seem that it would have no nutrients.

THE FACTS: Before it is roasted, a coffee bean contains the highest-known concentration of antioxidants of any food, and anti-oxidants play a big part in helping to prevent cell damage and inflam-

Before it is roasted, a coffee bean contains the highest-known concentration of antioxidants of any food.

mation. Coffee is Americans' primary source of dietary antioxidants. Unfortunately, the roasting process diminishes these levels, so the exact amount of antioxidants in our cup depends on how the green coffee beans were processed, roasted, and brewed. Some manufacturers are trying new methods of roasting to preserve more of these antioxidants.

MYTH: Decaf is healthier.

WHY WE THINK THAT: Again, with the conflicting studies that are out there, some of us believe less caffeine in our system is better.

THE FACTS: "There is no significant difference in the antioxidant levels between decaf and regular coffee," says Joe Vinson, PhD, profes-sor of chemistry at the University of Scranton in Pennsylvania. "Increased roasting decreases antioxidants, but our data indicates that decaf coffee is only slightly lower in antioxidants than regular coffee from the same brand."

Jose Antonio, PhD, the CEO of the International Society of Sports Nutrition and co-author of *Javalution: Fitness and Weight Loss Through Functional Coffee,*[29] says even up to four cups per day of caffeinated coffee is a better choice than decaf, especially for enhanced exercise performance, energy, and weight loss. However, limit your consumption if you have high blood pressure and/or are sensitive to caffeine.

MYTH: Coffee is the main source of caffeine in America.

WHY WE THINK THAT: Coffee is the most popular drink in Amer-ica and it contains caffeine, so by association we think it is the main source of caffeine.

THE FACTS: Caffeine is found in many drinks besides coffee such as tea, cocoa, and some sodas.

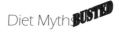

Table 6 shows a list of items that contain caffeine:

Table 6: Caffeine in popular drinks.[30]

Beverage	Caffeine
Coffee (10 oz.), brewed, drip	230 mg
Coffee (10 oz), instant	130 mg
Coffee (10 oz) decaf	5 mg
Tea (10 oz), brewed	80-120 mg
Iced tea (12 oz)	70 mg
Hot cocoa (8 oz)	5 mg
Coca-Cola (12 oz)	45 mg
Diet Coke (12 oz)	45 mg
Pepsi (12 oz)	40 mg
Diet Pepsi (12 oz)	40 mg
Dr. Pepper (12 oz)	40 mg
Mountain Dew (12 oz)	55 mg
Anacin (2 tablets)	32 mg
Excedrin (1 tablet)	65 mg
No-Doz (1 tablet)	100 mg
Red Bull (8.2 oz)	80 mg

MYTH: Coffee leads to heart disease.

WHY WE THINK THAT: Since coffee contains caffeine, we think that it will cause our heart rate and blood pressure to rise.

THE FACTS: Since coffee is a stimulant, it was believed it would lead to various forms of heart disease. A major study conducted by Willet, et al. examined data collected from more than 85,000 women over a ten-year period.[31] After adjusting the data for known risk factors, such as smoking, they found no increased risk of cardiovascular disease for women who drank six or more cups of coffee per day. A 1990 study by Grobbee, et al. found no link between coffee, caffeine, and cardiovascular disease in 45,000 men who drank four or more cups of coffee per day.[32]

Despite previous controversy on the subject, scientists now agree that regular caffeine use has little or no effect on blood pressure, cholesterol levels, or the risk of heart disease.

Studies show that while first-time users of caffeine experience a slight increase in blood pressure similar to that experienced when walking up stairs, the changes are minimal and disappear with regular use.

Regular caffeine use has little or no effect on blood pressure, cholesterol levels, or the risk of heart disease.

It has also been found that only boiled, unfiltered coffee, such as that taken in some Scandinavian countries, elevates cholesterol.[33] It seems the oils in the coffee that are not filtered out are responsible for this effect, not the coffee or caffeine. Consumption of caffeine-containing beverages does not typically affect cholesterol levels.

MYTH: Coffee causes ulcers.

WHY WE THINK THAT: Since coffee stains teeth and porous dishes, it appears corrosive, so we think it causes ulcers. Also, if we have an ulcer that we are unaware of and drink coffee, it may hurt, and we may think the coffee caused the ulcer instead of the ulcerated area being irritated by the beverage.

THE FACTS: Most ulcers are caused by the bacteria *Helicobacter pylori* and can be cured with antibiotics. An important distinction to make is that although coffee or spicy foods don't cause ulcers, they can aggravate existing ulcers.

MYTH: The effects of caffeine are addictive.

WHY WE THINK THAT: Caffeine is a stimulant, stimulants are drugs, and drugs can be addictive, thus we think that caffeine is addictive.

THE FACTS: We are "addicted" to caffeine the way we are "addicted" to shopping, working, or television. The word "addiction" refers to a strong dependence on a drug characterized by severe withdrawal symptoms, tolerance leading to a need for higher doses, and loss of control with the need to consume more and more of the substance at any cost. Addicts tend to exhibit antisocial behavior and commit crimes to subsidize their habit.

Consumers of caffeine-containing beverages do not fall into this category. The *Diagnostic and Statistical Manual for Mental Disorders — Text Revision* does not list caffeine as an addictive substance. According to the World Health Organization, "There is no evidence whatsoever that caffeine use has even remotely comparable physical and social consequences which are associated with serious drugs of abuse."[34]

Caffeine is a mild stimulant, and therefore is considered a drug, but those who use caffeine don't have control problems, and most can reduce or stop using caffeine without any significant problems.

MYTH: Caffeine is a risk factor for osteoporosis.

WHY WE THINK THAT: We have read that caffeine leaches calcium from our bones, so we believe it must be a risk factor.

THE FACTS: Risk factors for osteoporosis are insufficient dietary calcium and vitamin D, excessively high-protein diets, smoking, the onset of menopause, low estrogen levels, low body weight, and a lack of physical activity. Several well-controlled studies have concluded that consuming moderate amounts of caffeine does not increase the risk of developing osteoporosis. A 1994 National Institutes of Health Consensus Statement on optimal bone health does not list caffeine among the risk factors which modify calcium balance and influence bone mass.[35] A study by the Pennsylvania State Medical School found that lifetime consumption of caffeine had no effect on bone density in 188 post-menopausal women.[36]

Consumption of caffeine does cause a small amount of calcium to be lost in the urine, so nutritionists recommend that women who drink five or more cups of coffee a day

Consuming moderate amounts of caffeine does not increase the risk of developing osteoporosis.

add milk to their coffee, and drink one extra glass of milk daily or take a calcium supplement.

MYTH: Caffeine causes cancer.

WHY WE THINK THAT: For a long time, caffeine had a bad reputation as an addictive substance, and we have been conditioned to think of addictive substances as causing cancer.

THE FACTS: The American Cancer Society takes the position that "available information does not suggest a recommendation against the moderate use of coffee. There is no indication that caffeine, a natural component of both coffee and tea, is a risk factor in human cancer."[37]

Scientific evidence shows that caffeine is not a risk factor for cancer. Two studies involving large numbers of people in Norway and Hawaii found no connection between developing cancer and regular coffee consumption.[38] Two separate studies conducted on caffeine use in Japan and in Germany found no link between caffeine consumption and the incidence of cancer.[39]

> *Caffeine is not a risk factor for cancer.*

MYTH: Caffeine adversely affects the health of children.

WHY WE THINK THAT: A few decades ago, people thought caffeine would stunt children's growth because it elevated their blood pressure. When I was a child, an elderly woman who was my babysitter caught her young son drinking coffee, and was so intent on stopping him because she feared it would affect his growth that, one night while he slept, she painted his stomach brown in an effort to scare him away from drinking coffee.

THE FACTS: Soft drinks and tea are the primary sources of caffeine that children consume, and children consume less caffeine than adults. Children process caffeine the same way as adults. Studies have shown that, when taken in moderate amounts, foods and drinks containing caffeine have no detectable effects on activity levels or attention spans in children.

MYTH: Energy drinks and caffeine burn calories.

WHY WE THINK THAT: Since caffeine elevates our heart rate, we believe we will burn more calories. We want to emulate the athletic people who are often shown on the energy drink's package, thus we believe the advertisements.

THE FACTS: Energy drinks are extremely popular, and most consumers aren't aware that these drinks rely on large doses of caffeine to give us that boost of energy.

> *Energy drinks rely on large doses of caffeine to give us that boost of energy.*

They are designed to give the user a false energy supply. The sugar in the drinks provides energy to push through exercise or performance but result in a crash at the end. During the use you can burn calories, but there has to be activity to do so. Red Bull, for example, has 110 calories and 27 grams of sugar. Other types of energy drinks are sugar free and don't provide much energy.

MYTH: Caffeinated drinks cause dehydration.

WHY WE THINK THAT: Health and exercise experts have warned for years that consuming caffeine and caffeinated beverages cause dehydration.

THE FACTS: Dr. Lawrence Armstrong, a professor of exercise and environmental physiology at the University of Connecticut, found that caffeine does not cause dehydration and is no more of a diuretic than water.

"While there have been several studies done that show caffeine is a mild diuretic, there is no evidence that exercise, when combined with

> *Caffeine does not cause dehydration*

the consumption of caffeine or caffeinated beverages, will result in chronic dehydration, and this is contrary to the advice of most exercise physiologists, physicians and dietitians," explains Armstrong, who has conducted fluid-balance research since 1980.

Armstrong's analysis of the scientific literature, focusing on moderate use of caffeine (equivalent to one to four cups of coffee a day), revealed:

- When consuming a caffeinated beverage, the body retains some of the fluid.

- Moderate caffeine consumption causes a mild diuresis very similar to that caused by water which, when consumed in large volume, increases urine output.
- A person who regularly consumes caffeine has a higher tolerance to the diuretic effect.
- There is no evidence that consumption of caffeinated beverages causes a fluid-electrolyte imbalance detrimental to health or exercise performance.

In a review article, Dr. Heinz Valtin noted that research has clearly shown that caffeinated beverages may be counted toward a person's daily fluid intake.

MYTH: Caffeine stimulates the appetite and should be avoided by those trying to lose weight.

WHY WE THINK THAT: We believe what we read in magazines and newspapers.

THE FACTS: Caffeine has never been scientifically proven to be an appetite stimulant.

MYTH: Tea contains more caffeine than coffee.

WHY WE THINK THAT: We have been told that or read that.

THE FACTS: On the contrary, tea contains far less caffeine than coffee. Here is a listing of various drinks and their caffeine levels:

Tea contains far less caffeine than coffee.

- Regular or diet cola: 11-70 mg per 12-ounce can
- Tea: 50 mg per 6.5-ounce cup
- Instant Coffee: 75 mg per 6.5-ounce cup
- Brewed (filtered/percolated) coffee: 100-115 mg per 6.5-ounce cup

MYTH: Herbal teas are a healthy alternative to black teas.

WHY WE THINK THAT: We think of black tea as commercial tea, as opposed to herbal tea, which we believe is a healthier option.

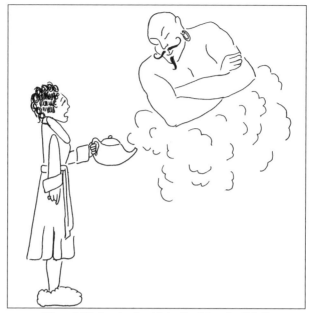

Harold? Just what kind of tea is this?

THE FACTS: Not necessarily. All teas are rich in powerful antioxidants called flavonoids. Increasing evidence shows that antioxidants found in tea, fruit, and vegetables are an important part of a healthy diet. Many herbal infusions contain pharmacologically active ingredients and antioxidants that are claimed to have positive benefits, but these claims are unsubstantiated. Recent research has shown that antioxidant levels in black tea are substantially greater than those in most herbal infusions, and that one or two cups of black tea can provide an antioxidant effect similar to five portions of fruit or vegetables or 400 mg of vitamin C.

MYTH: Green tea is a healthier alternative than black tea.

WHY WE THINK THAT: We tend to believe that black tea is more processed than green tea, so we think that green tea is healthier.

THE FACTS: Green and black teas both contain similar amounts of flavonoid components which differ only in their nature. Green tea contains proportionally more of the simple flavonoids called catechins while black tea mainly contains more complex flavonoids called theaflavins and thearubigins. Both the simple and complex flavonoids are powerful antioxidants that may reduce the risk of heart disease, stroke, and cancers. So drink both!

MYTH: The antioxidants in tea have little biological activity.

WHY WE THINK THAT: We tend to believe that fruits and vegetables have more antioxidants than tea.

THE FACTS: Research shows that antioxidants may have a protective role to play in certain conditions such as heart disease, stroke, and cancers. It is well known that fruits and vegetables are good

> *Every time you use a tea bag to brew a cup or a pot of tea, you are drinking about 140 mg of flavonoids.*

sources of antioxidants. Three cups of tea contain eight times the amount of "antioxidant power" found in one apple. Every time you use a tea bag to brew a cup or a pot of tea, you are drinking about 140 mg of flavonoids.

MYTH: Tea is bad for our teeth because it stains them.

WHY WE THINK THAT: Our teeth are porous, and both coffee and tea produce stains when the teeth are not brushed.

THE FACTS: On the contrary, recent research suggests that flavonoids and fluoride in tea may actually be beneficial to teeth by reducing cavities and helping to prevent plaque from developing. As long as teeth are brushed regularly, stains will not occur.

MYTH: Tea is a diuretic and causes dehydration.

WHY WE THINK THAT: The same experts who told us coffee was a diuretic also said the same about tea due to the caffeine content.

THE FACTS: Tea does not have a diuretic effect due to caffeine, unless a person drinks an enormous amount. The diuretic effect of tea is the same as that of coffee. Drinking a lot of any liquid will have a diuretic effect on anyone. The British Dietetic Association advises that tea, like coffee, juice, milk, and water, can contribute towards the normal intake of fluids.[40]

MYTH: Adding milk to tea reduces the antioxidant activity.

WHY WE THINK THAT: A recent sound bite claimed that adding milk or cream to our tea nullified the health benefits of tea.

THE FACTS: Studies have found that the flavonoids in tea are absorbed equally well from tea with and without milk. The addition of milk did not affect the body's ability to absorb and use these antioxidants.

> *The flavonoids in tea are absorbed equally well from tea with and without milk.*

MYTH: Green tea is a miracle fat-burner.

WHY WE THINK THAT: Many popular magazines have advertisements for weight-loss pills and drinks that contain green tea.

THE FACTS: Green tea, or any tea, does not cause your body to burn large amounts of fat. If there is an increase in your metabolism from green tea, it is very small, even if you take multiple doses of green tea each day, because your body adapts to this. Drinking tea is a good choice because it is free of sugar and calories. So drink it for its other health benefits, not because someone told you that it'll help you lose weight fast!

MYTH: Green tea prevents cancer.

WHY WE THINK THAT: Green tea, as well as certain fruits and vegetables, has been marketed as a cure for cancer, and we want to believe this.

THE FACTS: Tea has antioxidant properties but these are not enough to prevent prostate and other cancers. The consumption of green tea as an anticancer measure has not won FDA approval. The National Cancer Institute recently studied 42 prostate-cancer patients who drank about four cups of green tea daily for four months. Only one patient experienced a short-lived improvement. Seventy percent of the group experienced unpleasant side effects, such as nausea and diarrhea, but did not experience significant improvement. The study concluded that drinking green tea has limited antitumor benefit for prostate-cancer patients.[41]

Important rule of thumb: Avoid holiday-themed items from coffee shops at all costs. From peppermint to eggnog to pumpkin, these are often the most sugar and calorie-packed drinks you'll find at Starbucks and other coffee shops.

Hot coffee to avoid: Starbucks Venti 2% Peppermint White Chocolate Mocha: 660 calories, 22 grams of fat (14 grams saturated), 95 grams of sugar. Other coffee shops have similar diet-busting blends.

Frozen coffee drink to avoid: Cosi Gigante Double OH! Arctic (24 ounces): 1,033 calories, 35 grams of fat, 177 grams of carbohydrates.

Frozen coffee concoctions dilute the antioxidant powers of a simple cup of regular coffee with a huge hit of fats, sugary syrups, and whipped cream. What you get in worst-case scenarios like this is half a day's worth of empty calories, ready to be sipped down in a matter of minutes. There are lots of other choices to avoid, too. Want a cold caffeine kick? Try iced coffee.

What to take away

- Coffee and tea are not diuretics and don't cause dehydration.
- Both coffee and tea contain antioxidants, but not enough to be a medical cure for anything.
- Caffeine is not a harmful substance and, if taken in moderation, has many positive benefits.

13. ALCOHOL

You can't be a real country unless you have a beer and an airline
— it helps if you have some kind of a football team, or some
nuclear weapons, but at the very least you need a beer.
— Frank Zappa

Our body needs a set number of calories to maintain our weight. This need is based on height, weight, age, gender, and activity level. When we consume more calories than our body needs, we gain weight. Alcohol contains many calories in a small volume and can be a source of unwanted extra calories when consumed in excess, thus causing weight gain.

Studies have shown that in the short term alcohol stimulates the appetite and can also increase feelings of hunger. Other studies

> When we consume alcohol, we consume more food.

have shown that the stimulatory effects of alcohol on food intake are controlled by hormonal regulation of satiation, such as by the hormone leptin. Regardless of the cause, the outcome is the same: when we consume alcohol, we consume more food. One study showed when we drink alcohol before a meal, we increase our calorie consumption at the meal by 20%. This created a total caloric increase of 33% when the calories from the alcohol were added, and can easily contribute to weight gain over a short amount of time.

Regulating our calorie consumption is the key to successful weight loss and maintenance. A balanced diet will curb our hunger and provide the necessary nutrients for health and wellness. Alcohol is not considered a necessary component of a healthy diet. As we start changing our eating habits, eliminating alcohol is recommended. Once we have established new, healthy eating habits, alcohol can be added back to our diet in limited quantities, if desired.

We have to count the calories from alcohol in any diet plan. Calories from alcoholic drinks can be limited by choosing those with less alcohol and by consuming a limited amount of sweetened beverages. We can also use flavored seltzers or water to dilute the alcohol so we will consume fewer calories. Another helpful tip to consume less alcohol is to sip our drinks over a long period of time.

When consumed in excess, alcohol adds a lot of calories to our diet and negatively impacts many aspects of our health. If we choose to consume alcohol, we need to limit the quantity and frequency. Table 7 shows the calorie contents for some common alcoholic drinks.

> *If we choose to consume alcohol, we need to limit the quantity and frequency.*

Alcohol contains calories but, paradoxically, according to extensive medical research, drinking alcohol without also consuming food doesn't lead to weight gain, and many studies report a small reduction in weight for women who drink. The reason that alcohol alone doesn't increase weight is unclear, but research suggests that energy from alcohol is not efficiently used. Alcohol also appears to increase metabolic rate significantly, thus causing more calories to be burned rather than stored in the body as fat. Other research has found that sugar consumption decreases as consumption of alcohol increases. But drinking only alcohol and not eating is not a healthy way of losing weight!

Whatever the reasons, the consumption of alcohol in moderation is

Table 7: Calorie content for selected alcoholic drinks.

Alcoholic Drink	Calories
Beer, lite, 12 oz.	100
Beer, regular, 12 oz.	150
Frozen daiquiri, 4 oz.	216
Gin, 1½ oz.	110
Mai tai, 4 oz.	310
Margarita, 4 oz.	270
Rum, 1½ oz.	96
Vodka, 1½ oz.	96
Whiskey, 1½ oz.	105
Wine spritzer, 4 oz.	49
Wine, dessert, sweet, 4 oz.	180

not associated with weight gain and is often associated with weight loss in women. The medical evidence for this is based on a large number of studies of thousands of people around the world. Some of these studies are very large; one such study involved nearly 80,000 women and another included 140,000 subjects.[42] Alcoholic beverages contain no fat, no cholesterol, and very little sodium. Of course, the nutritional value of different alcohol beverages varies. Moderate consumption of alcohol is associated with better health and longer life compared to either abstaining from alcohol or abusing alcohol. However, any health benefits of drinking are evident only when consumed in moderation. Heavy drinking is associated with cirrhosis of the liver, breast cancer, and other serious health problems. The key word is moderation.

In the United States moderation is often described as two drinks a day for a man and one drink a day for a woman. These drinks can't be "saved up" over time and then consumed in one day. One drink is:

> *Moderate consumption of alcohol is associated with better health and longer life compared to either abstaining from alcohol or abusing alcohol.*

- 12-ounce bottle or can of regular beer
- six-ounce glass of dinner wine
- shot of liquor or spirits, either straight or in a mixed drink

Remember that the alcohol content of standard drinks is equivalent. A drink is a drink is a drink. To a breathalyzer and a traffic cop, they're all the same.

Now for the myths:

MYTH: All alcohol is bad for you.

WHY WE THINK THAT: A lot of bad things can happen when alcohol is abused. We tend to dwell on the negatives and not the positives.

THE FACTS: Alcohol is an anticoagulant. Red wine contains antioxidants, so drinking a small amount can be beneficial. Moderation is the key when it comes to alcohol. Moderate amounts of alcohol for the average adult are 1½ ounces of hard liquor, six ounces of wine, or 12 ounces of beer per day.

MYTH: Alcohol destroys brain cells.

WHY WE THINK THAT: Although legal, alcohol is considered a drug, and we tend to associate drug use with negative effects. Too much alcohol negatively affects people in many ways, including their ability to think rationally.

THE FACTS: The moderate consumption of alcohol does not destroy brain cells. In fact, it is often associated with improved cognitive functioning. However, consistent abuse of alcohol will cause blackouts and brain deterioration.

> *Moderate consumption of alcohol is often associated with improved cognitive functioning.*

MYTH: Hard liquor has a higher alcohol content and therefore has a higher calorie content.

WHY WE THINK THAT: Hard liquor tends to have a hard-biting taste when consumed straight, and a small volume packs the same alcoholic punch as a bottle of beer or a glass of wine, so we assume it has more calories.

THE FACTS: One serving, 1½ ounce of any 80-proof hard liquor, has 100 calories. If it is 100-proof, the calorie content is 124 calories. A 6-ounce glass of wine has 120 calories, a 6.5-ounce flute of champagne has 163 calories, and a 12-ounce bottle of beer has 150 calories. Since 1½ ounce of liquor is a smaller volume than a bottle of beer or glass of wine, it is easier to drink more and thus accumulate more calories.

MYTH: A beer belly is caused by drinking beer.

WHY WE THINK THAT: We believe what we see. Many people who have paunches also drink a lot of beer, so we put the two together.

THE FACTS: A beer belly is caused by eating too much food and drinking too many calorie-dense beverages, whether they are alcoholic or non-alcoholic drinks. While beer or other alcoholic beverages will add additional calories, they are not the only culprits. However, overconsumption of alcohol will make a "six pack" become a "keg!"

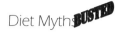

MYTH: White wine is a good choice for a person who wants a light drink with less alcohol.

WHY WE THINK THAT: We tend to associate a lighter color and a less pungent taste with less effect.

THE FACTS: A standard drink, whether a glass of white or red wine, a bottle of beer, a shot of whiskey or other distilled spirits, contains equal amounts of alcohol. All forms of alcoholic beverage are the same to a Breathalyzer.

All forms of alcoholic beverage are the same to a Breathalyzer.

MYTH: Drinking wine instead of beer won't give you a beer belly.

WHY WE THINK THAT: We associate drinking beer with men who have a large belly and watch NASCAR and drinking wine with sophisticated slender types who attend cheese-tasting events at museums.

THE FACTS: A common misconception is that wine contains fewer calories than beer. A six-ounce glass of wine contains 120 calories compared to a 12-ounce bottle of beer, which has 150 calories. Therefore, ounce for ounce, wine actually has more calories, and sweeter wine has even more sugar and calories. So, even though they drink only wine, a person can still get a "beer belly" if they overconsume.

MYTH: Switching between beer, wine, and spirits will lead to intoxication more quickly than sticking to one type of alcoholic beverage.

WHY WE THINK THAT: By switching between different types of drinks, we run the risk of drinking too much and thus we assume that it is the drinking of different types of alcohol, rather than the amount, that causes intoxication.

THE FACTS: The level of blood alcohol determines sobriety or intoxication, no matter where the alcohol comes from. Remember that a standard drink of beer, wine, or spirits contains the same amount of alcohol. Alcohol is alcohol and a drink is a drink. If mixing drinks were really a problem, restaurants wouldn't be able to serve a cocktail before dinner, wine with dinner, and an after-dinner drink to patrons.

MYTH: Drinking coffee will help an intoxicated person become sober.

WHY WE THINK THAT: We see it in the movies and have heard that coffee sobers a person up, so we think it must work.

THE FACTS: Only time will make a person sober, not black coffee, cold showers, exercise, or any other common "cures." Alcohol leaves the blood and, therefore, the body at a constant rate of about

> Only time will make a person sober. (A cold shower makes a drunk person a very awake, wet, cold, drunk person.)

0.015% per hour. A person with a blood alcohol content (BAC) of 0.015 would be completely sober in an hour while a person with a BAC of ten times that (0.15) requires 10 hours to become completely sober. This is true regardless of sex, age, or weight. The only thing coffee does is make a drunk person a very awake, drunk person, and a cold shower makes a drunk person a very awake, wet, cold, drunk person.

MYTH: Drinking over a long period of time will cause a person to become an alcoholic.

WHY WE THINK THAT: We assume if a person drinks over a life-time, they must need to drink rather than want to drink.

THE FACTS: There is simply no scientific basis for this misperception. It originates from old temperance and prohibitionist ideology. A distinction also needs to be made between alcoholism and alcohol abuse. They are not the same. An alcoholic usually abuses alcohol. An abuser of alcohol may not be an alcoholic. Alcoholism is determined by a person's dependency on alcohol, how much a person drinks at a time, if it is the center of the person's life, and if it controls the person actions. Not distinguishing between alcohol abuse and alcoholism has led to much confusion about why some people can easily step away from drinking and others can't.

I have known people who enjoy drinking and do so almost every day, and yet never abuse alcohol. They have one or two drinks and are particular about their choices. I have also known people who don't drink for days at a time, usually during the workweek, but when the weekend comes and they do drink, they abuse alcohol and drink to excess each

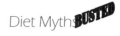

and every time and it doesn't matter to them where the alcohol comes from. Some abuse alcohol by drinking a lot, every day, all day. What we do know from research is that moderate use of alcohol (except, perhaps, for pregnant women) is healthier than alcohol abuse and also non-use of alcohol.

MYTH: Drunkenness and alcoholism are the same thing.

WHY WE THINK THAT: When we see someone who is drunk, we assume they may have a problem with alcohol.

THE FACTS: Many non-alco-holics on occasion become intoxi-cated or drunk. However, if they are not addicted to alcohol, they are not alcoholic. Of course, intoxication is

It is better either to abstain or to drink moderately than to overindulge.

never completely safe or risk-free, and should be avoided. It is better either to abstain or to drink moderately than to overindulge. While con-suming alcohol sensibly is associated with better health and longer life, the abuse of alcohol is associated with many undesirable health out-comes.

MYTH: Drinking alcohol causes weight gain.

WHY WE THINK THAT: This is a very commonly believed myth, even among medical professionals, because alcohol contains seven calories per gram.

THE FACTS: Extensive research around the world has found that al-cohol consumption alone does not cause weight gain in men and is often associated with a small amount of weight loss in women. Alcohol, like any other food or drink, will cause weight gain if it is part of a diet that provides more calories than a person burns off through physical activity.

MYTH: Men and women of the same height and weight can drink the same amount.

WHY WE THINK THAT: We have been told over and over that how much a person weighs determines how alcohol will affect them. It is natural to assume that if a man and a woman weigh the same, alcohol will affect them the same.

THE FACTS: Women are affected more rapidly because they tend to have a slightly higher proportion of fat to lean muscle tissue, thus concentrating alcohol a little more easily, since alcohol tends to collect in fat. Women also have less of an enzyme (alcohol dehydrogenase) that metabolizes (breaks down) alcohol. Hormonal changes during their menstrual cycle may also affect alcohol absorption to some degree.

MYTH: A single sip of alcohol by a pregnant woman can cause her child to have fetal alcohol syndrome (FAS).

WHY WE THINK THAT: We all know that excessive alcohol consumption is bad for a fetus, so we assume any alcohol is bad.

THE FACTS: Extensive medical research studying hundreds of thousands of women from around the world has not found any scientific evidence that light drinking, much less a single sip of alcohol, by an expectant mother can cause fetal alcohol syndrome. Of course, the very safest choice is to abstain from alcohol throughout pregnancy. However, many expectant mothers drink responsibly and socially before they are aware they are pregnant. Once aware of their condition, it would be prudent to abstain from alcohol as the safest option, but there is no need to feel guilty about having a drink before knowing one's condition.

MYTH: People who abstain from alcohol are "alcohol-free."

WHY WE THINK THAT: We assume that unless we consume something, it does not reside in us through other means.

THE FACTS: Every person's body produces a small amount of alcohol 24 hours a day from birth until death. Therefore, we always have some alcohol in our bodies.

> *Every person's body produces a small amount of alcohol.*

MYTH: Bottles of tequila contain a worm.

WHY WE THINK THAT: We have all seen the worm in the bottle. Customarily, when passing around the bottle, the person who ends up with the last swig has to eat the worm.

THE FACTS: Bottles of tequila don't all contain a worm. Those that have the "worm" actually contain a "gusano," the larval form of the

Hipopta agavis moth that lives on the agave plants from which tequila is distilled. If one of these "gusanos" is found in your bottle of tequila, some say it indicates an inferior-quality product. Some also say that the gusano was added to bottles of mescal, an alcoholic beverage made in the Mexican state of Oaxaca and also distilled from agave, as a marketing gimmick. Whatever the true story is, I still wouldn't want to eat the "worm."

MYTH: People who can "hold their liquor" are to be envied.

WHY WE THINK THAT: When we see someone who appears able to drink a lot of alcohol without showing any signs of drunkenness, we envy them because they can indulge while the rest of us must be more cautious and limit our intake.

THE FACTS: People who can drink heavily without becoming intoxicated have probably developed a tolerance for alcohol, which can indicate the onset of dependency, or alcoholism. Overconsumption leads to an increased appetite, which leads to overconsumption of both food and drink, leading to weight gain and a loss of physical fitness. This is not an enviable position. While studies have indicated that alcohol consumption doesn't lead to weight gain, the studies are based on moderate intake, not overindulgence.

MYTH: Alcohol is the cause of alcoholism.

WHY WE THINK THAT: Since alcoholics drink alcohol to excess we assume alcohol is the cause.

THE FACTS: There are many factors involved in alcoholism, including patterns of alcohol use. These are the cause of alcoholism rather than alcohol itself according to the U. S. National Institutes of Health.

There are many factors involved in alcoholism, including patterns of alcohol use.

A common belief among members of Alcoholics Anonymous (AA) is that people are born with a genetic predisposition to be alcoholic. They do not become alcoholic because of alcohol or anything else in their experience. AA argues that some people can be born and die as alcoholics without ever having had a sip of alcohol. Of course, a person can't be

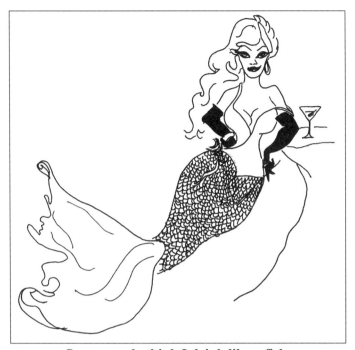

Some people think I drink like a fish.

a "practicing alcoholic" without consuming alcohol. The evidence is not clearly in favor of any position.

Trying to keep people completely away from alcohol through Prohibition led to problems: an increase in heavy drinking, death and disability from contaminated illegal alcohol, growth of organized crime, loss of tax revenue, the discouragement of moderate consumption, disrespect for the law, and other social ills. Therefore, if we choose to drink we must do so responsibly. If we are not able to drink responsibly, it is better not to drink at all.

Cocktail to avoid: Piña Colada, 625 calories, 75 grams of sugar. Made from a blend of sweet pineapple juice and fatty coconut milk, piña coladas may be one of the biggest saboteurs for anyone wanting to sport a bikini. In fact, the only redeeming part of this drink, besides its fantastic taste, is the chunk of pineapple hanging from the rim. Try a lime daiquiri or a mojito instead, and save up to 400 calories a drink.

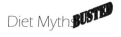

What to take away

- Alcohol can be beneficial or detrimental to us, depending on how we consume it.
- When part of a healthy lifestyle and consumed in moderation, alcohol will not cause excessive weight gain.
- When consumed in excess and abused, alcohol will cause weight gain, brain damage, liver damage, and dependency.

14. CHOLESTEROL — A NECESSARY FAT

As for butter versus margarine, I trust cows more than chemists.
— Joan Gussow

If I'd known I was going to live this long, I'd have taken better care of myself.
— Eubie Blake (On his 100th Birthday)

Cholesterol is a biologically necessary fat that is manufactured by our bodies. Sunlight and natural chemical reactions in our bodies convert it into Vitamin D, and it's the precursor for steroid hormones, such as testosterone, estrogen, and some of the adrenal gland hormones, which are necessary for normal growth and development of our bodies.

Even when we don't consume any cholesterol at all, our liver manufactures around 1,000 milligrams (mg) of cholesterol every day. About 80% of this becomes

> Cholesterol is a biologically necessary fat that is manufactured by our bodies.

bile salts, which are necessary for the digestion of fats, leaving about 200 mg available for other functions.

When our diet contains cholesterol, the liver simply makes less of it. The typical American diet contains 250-350 mg per day, but only a third to half of that is absorbed, or about 85-175 mg, so out of that 1,000 mg of cholesterol in the liver, only 10%-15% comes from our diet. Even if we eliminate cholesterol from the diet, a healthy person's liver makes more to make up for the deficit. Eliminating saturated fat from our diet doesn't change anything either, because the liver will make cholesterol out of sugar and starch. That's how necessary and important cholesterol is to our body. When the liver isn't functioning well, dietary intake of cholesterol becomes essential. A study at the University of California — Berkeley found that dietary cholesterol improved the mental ability of people facing advancing age and declining memory.[43]

Dietary intake of cholesterol is not the cause of high cholesterol. So what is? If our liver behaves as if the cholesterol it has manufactured has been used up when it actually is still present, our cholesterol levels rise. In the past, when we were always on the move, looking for food, and doing physical labor to build our homes and acquire supplies and food, the liver never had this problem because it kept supplying cholesterol, which was constantly being used up by our physically active lives. But now, even though most of us live a sedentary lifestyle, our metabolism is still based on a body that was constantly active doing physical work. The result is our liver makes an oversupply of cholesterol that our body does not use up.

Even though the cholesterol and saturated fat in our diet are not responsible for high cholesterol levels, that doesn't give us license

There are two forms of cholesterol; oxidized and unoxidized.

to go out and eat all the high-cholesterol, fatty foods we want. The quality of the fat in our food is critical to maintain adequate cholesterol levels as well as overall good health. It turns out that there are two forms of cholesterol; oxidized and unoxidized. Our livers only make the unoxidized form. Only oxidized cholesterol causes coronary heart disease and the only source of oxidized cholesterol is our food. When cholesterol is exposed to sunlight, oxygen, or heat, it is oxidized in a way similar to how oils are hydrogenated or superheated to make trans fats. This oxidation can happen in clear bottles stored on shelves exposed to light or by exposure to free radicals that have come into our bodies from unhealthy foods, especially foods containing trans fats, since free radicals can be created in similarly stored, commercially processed oils. When we consume commercially processed oils, the cholesterol in our body can be oxidized by the free radicals found in those oils.

Although refined and hydrogenated oils have been deodorized to remove their smell, they're still rancid and contain an unknown amount of oxidized cholesterol. Some people with high cholesterol levels never have a heart attack because none of their cholesterol is oxidized. Others, even with normal or low levels of cholesterol, have heart attacks because much of their cholesterol is oxidized. There is simply no connection between unoxidized cholesterol levels and heart attacks. After monitoring 5,000 people for several decades, the Framingham Heart Study determined that people who eat cholesterol from unprocessed sources do not have an increased risk of developing coronary heart disease. Meanwhile, a study at Albany Medical College showed that "pure unadulterated cholesterol is not harmful to the arteries and cannot initiate or promote heart disease."[44]

Let's look at the myths.

MYTH: Eating foods containing cholesterol will raise our blood cholesterol level.

WHY WE THINK THAT: We have been told that eating foods containing cholesterol is bad and will raise our cholesterol. We are bombarded with advertisements for numerous drugs that are meant to lower our cholesterol, so we believe cholesterol is bad. We think of arteries as pipes and cholesterol as gooey, sticky gunk. We think if we eat cholesterol, it winds up in our blood. We think if the cholesterol level in our blood gets too high, it will clog up the pipes. Therefore, if we don't want our pipes clogged, we don't eat foods rich in cholesterol. That's the logic behind the advice to avoid eating nutrient-dense foods, such as liver and egg yolks.

People who eat cholesterol from unprocessed sources do not have an increased risk of developing coronary heart disease.

FACTS: The average person's liver makes 75% or more of their cholesterol and the other 25% or so comes from food. The more a person exercises, the more HDL (good) cholesterol their body will make, since HDL is a substance that the body uses. Most of us can't eat any more cholesterol than we can use. If we avoid foods with cholesterol, our body will just produce what we need. There is no direct connection between the amount of cholesterol we eat and the concentration of cholesterol in our blood. In most people, eating cholesterol has little or no effect on this amount. In about 30% of the population, eating choles-

There is no direct connection between the amount of cholesterol we eat and the concentration of cholesterol in our blood.

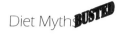

terol does in fact increase the concentration of cholesterol in the blood, but it increases the "good" HDL cholesterol.

MYTH: Total blood serum cholesterol should be 200 mg/dl or less.
WHY WE THINK THAT: For decades we have been told that we should have a total cholesterol level of no more than 200 mg/dl or we will increase our risk of heart disease.

FACTS: Individuals with total cholesterol levels lower than 200 mg/dl actually have a higher death rate from heart disease. Cholesterol

Cholesterol ratios are more important than the overall number.

ratios are more important than the overall number. As long as the HDL is 40 mg/dl or higher for men and 50 mg/dl or higher for women, and the LDL is 150 mg/dl or lower for men and women alike, the levels are good. My total cholesterol level is 234 mg/dl, my HDL is 125 mg/dl, and my LDL is 109 mg/dl. Since I am physically very active, my higher cholesterol level is okay because my body uses what it makes. And even though my overall cholesterol level looks high, my cholesterol is excellent because my HDL is very high and my LDL is lower with a ratio of total cholesterol to HDL of about 1.9. Anything less than 4.5 is considered good; 1.9 is excellent.

Research consistently shows that dietary cholesterol intake does not increase blood cholesterol or a person's cardiac risk. Because the body makes its own cholesterol, eating more means that the body will produce less, and eating less means that the body will produce more. Only a small percentage of the population doesn't regulate blood cholesterol well, and they will have high cholesterol regardless of dietary intake. The best way to deal with concerns about blood cholesterol is to increase activity through exercise, and improve the quality of our overall diet, not vilify foods that contain cholesterol.

In a recent review, cholesterol researcher Dr. Maria Luz Fernandez of the University of Connecticut's Department of Nutritional Sciences summarized the results of a number of studies that looked at the effects of egg consumption on blood cholesterol levels.[45] In children aged 10-12 years, in men aged 20-50, in premenopausal and postmenopausal women, and in Caucasians and Hispanics, the same basic finding persisted: eating two to three eggs a day has little or no effect on the blood cholesterol levels of over two-thirds of the population.

In contrast, less than a third of the population are *hyperresponders.* When hyperresponders eat egg yolks, their cholesterol levels go up, but their LDL and HDL go up equally, so there is no change in the ratio of LDL to HDL or of LDL to total cholesterol.

Moreover, the actual number of LDL particles does not change at all; they just get bigger. When your doctor measures your blood cholesterol level, the lab reports it by weight. In America, this is usually in milligrams (mg) per deciliter (dl). When your cholesterol level is high, this means that in a given volume of blood (such as a deciliter) the total number of cholesterol-carrying lipoprotein particles weighs more. This could mean that you have more particles or that the particles weigh more because they are carrying more cholesterol.

There are two types of LDL-cholesterol particles. Research has found that the small, dense LDL particles raise the risk of atherosclerosis while the large, buoyant LDL particles do not. This is because small, dense LDL particles are much more vulnerable to oxidation. People whose LDL is primarily small and dense have three times the risk of heart disease than people whose LDL is primarily large and buoyant. In studies where people consume eggs, the LDL particles get bigger, not more numerous. When they get bigger, they become less likely to oxidize and accumulate in atherosclerotic plaques.

If arteries were like pipes and cholesterol was like gunk, more gunk would just clog up the pipe, but arteries are nothing like pipes and cholesterol is nothing like gunk.

Arteries are nothing like pipes and cholesterol is nothing like gunk.

MYTH: Cholesterol is a dangerous fat.

WHY WE THINK THAT: For years, almost every doctor, nutritionist, and food advertisement has warned us about the evils of cholesterol. We have been told that cholesterol is the cause of accumulated plaque in our arteries and leads to heart disease. An entire industry revolves around measuring cholesterol levels, lowering cholesterol levels, and creating foods and drugs that we're told will make us healthier by lowering our cholesterol levels.

THE FACTS: Cholesterol is naturally made by the body. Nothing naturally made by the body is a bad thing unless it becomes imbalanced, and anything that is imbalanced can create symptoms that tell us to get back into balance. Cholesterol is an important nutrient that strengthens cell membranes and intestinal walls, is necessary to make bile, and is vital for hormone and vitamin production.

Cholesterol boosts our immune system and is an antioxidant that protects us from free radicals. Recent research suggests that diets high in cholesterol actually protect against neurodegenerative disorders such as Parkinson's and Alzheimer's diseases. Serotonin receptors in the brain need cholesterol to function properly, brain cells must last a lifetime, and cholesterol is a brain protector.

> Diets high in cholesterol actually protect against neurodegenerative disorders such as Parkinson's and Alzheimer's diseases.

MYTH: Heart disease is caused by the consumption of cholesterol and saturated fat in animal products.

WHY WE THINK THAT: Groups that we trust have told us that since fat is a dense, heavy food source, it will clog our arteries and give us heart disease.

THE FACTS: At the same time Dr. Ancel Keys was looking for facts to support his concept that saturated fats caused heart disease, another researcher, Dr. David Kritchevsky, was doing research on cholesterol and heart disease. Like Keys, Kritchevsky decided that cholesterol was harmful and engineered research to prove it. He force-fed rabbits purified cholesterol, which induced the growth of plaque in their arteries.[46] But rabbits do not naturally eat dairy products or meat, rabbits aren't made to eat or process fat, and the plaque induced in the rabbits' arteries was totally different from the plaque in human arteries.

Heart disease increased rapidly between 1920 and 1960, but at the same time the consumption of meat and animal fats declined. During this same time period, the consumption of hydrogenated and industrially processed vegetable fats (omega-6 oils) increased dramatically. The manufacturers of vegetable oils took advantage of the flawed research done by Keys and Kritchevsky and used it to push their oils onto the public, using slogans like "for your heart's sake." The ingestion of these oils has been more closely associated with heart disease than the consumption of saturated fats or foods that contain cholesterol.

MYTH: Abnormal cholesterol readings are caused by eating large amounts of fat.

WHY WE THINK THAT: Most of us have been taught that a high-fat diet causes cholesterol problems.

THE FACTS: The types of fat that we eat are more important than the amount of fat. Trans fats or hydrogenated fats and large amounts of saturated fats promote

> *The types of fat that we eat are more important than the amount of fat.*

abnormal cholesterol production. Omega-3 fats and monounsaturated fat improve the type and quantity of cholesterol produced by our bodies. In reality, the biggest source of abnormal cholesterol is not fat at all but sugar. When we consume too much sugar, it converts to fat in our body. The worst type of sugar is high-fructose corn syrup. Overconsumption of high-fructose corn syrup, which is present in sodas, many juices, and most processed foods, is the primary nutritional cause of most of the cholesterol issues doctors see in their patients.

MYTH: Cholesterol-reducing drugs save our lives.

WHY WE THINK THAT: That is what many doctors and advertisements tell us. We think we need to lower our cholesterol, and believe that cholesterol-lowering drugs do just that, thus saving our lives.

THE FACTS: Cholesterol-reducing drugs are the largest selling drugs in the world and they are produced and marketed in response to questionable science. Shutting down a critical nutrient like cholesterol has serious consequences, and the problems found to be caused by these drugs are far more wide reaching than first thought.

The lipid-lowering or cholesterol-reducing drugs have been increasingly implicated in a number of lymphatic cancers, neurological problems, and heart health issues, which are the very problems they were supposed to treat! The latest drug to fall from grace is the statin drug, Vytorin. Several studies have shown that statin drugs shut down coenzyme Q_{10} (CoQ_{10}), which has serious ramifications. Without CoQ_{10} we cannot produce ATP (adenosine triphosphate), which is the root energy source for our whole body, including the heart. Many people are already deficient in CoQ_{10} by the time they are over 50, the age group in which most heart attacks occur, and statins reduce CoQ_{10} by up to 40%. Low CoQ_{10} levels have also been implicated in other disorders, such as Parkinson's and Alzheimer's diseases.

MYTH: Cholesterol levels are the best indicator of potential heart problems or heart disease.

WHY WE THINK THAT: At a certain age we all regularly have our cholesterol levels checked, either at the doctor's office or at home using the new home test kits that are being recommended and sold in pharmacies throughout the world. We become convinced that if our overall cholesterol levels are high, we are at risk for heart problems.

THE FACTS: Our levels of C-reactive protein (CRP), homocysteine, and fasting blood sugar are far better indicators of our heart health, yet doctors who have been indoctrinated with the cholesterol myth are reluctant to use these tests. Our level of oxidized (damaged) LDL, which may indicate how healthy we are, actually reflects a shortage of antioxidants, not a need for statin drugs. A damaged form of LDL-cholesterol is found in powdered eggs, powdered milk, microwaved meats and fats, and in well-done steaks.

> *Our levels of C-reactive protein (CRP), homocysteine, and fasting blood sugar are the best indicators of our heart health.*

Our fasting blood sugar (glucose) level is one of the best indicators of heart health. If blood sugar is high, the risks of heart attack and stroke are increased by 500%. Elevated blood sugar stimulates the production of free radicals, reduces the uptake of the antioxidant vitamin C into our cells, impairs immune function, decreases the antioxidant nitric oxide in our arteries, inhibits the breakdown of clots, and dramatically increases glycation (non-enzymatic glycosylation), which is the bonding of sugar to protein molecules. This glyco-oxidation makes the collagen in the walls of our arteries less able to expand and contract, thus creating atherosclerosis, which attracts plaque like a magnet. In simple terms, elevated blood sugar is *the* risk factor for hardening of the arteries.

MYTH: Eating eggs will raise our cholesterol levels.

WHY WE THINK THAT: Eggs have been singled out as a high cholesterol-containing villain for a long time. This myth began because egg yolks contain the most concentrated amount of cholesterol of any food.

FACTS: There is not enough cholesterol in egg yolks to pose a health risk, if eggs are eaten in moderation. Studies suggest that

There is not enough cholesterol in egg yolks to pose a health risk.

eating one egg per day will not raise cholesterol levels, and that eating two or three eggs a day is safe in a balanced diet with adequate exercise. Eggs are actually a great source of nutrients and they are one of the best and least expensive foods on the planet.

MYTH: We should eat only the egg whites and throw away the egg yolks.

WHY WE THINK THAT: We believe that if we eat foods that contain cholesterol, we will increase our blood cholesterol levels and our risk of heart disease.

FACTS: Egg yolks have been vilified for a long time because they contain most of the fat in the egg. The fat in an egg is part cholesterol, part saturated fat, part monounsaturated fat, and is a good source of omega-3. The vitamin lecithin, which is good for the eyes, is also found in egg yolks.

MYTH: We should eat only the egg yolks and throw away the egg whites.

WHY WE THINK THAT: Some personal trainers and serious athletes claim that only the yolk of the egg is good for us, and that we should throw away the egg whites.

FACTS: Eggs are a complete food. Egg yolks have all of the required fat-soluble vitamins (A, D, E, and K), iron, and heart-healthy omega-3 fatty acids. The whites have all of the many water-soluble B vitamins and contain more than half of an egg's protein. Important minerals, such as chlorine, magnesium, potassium, sodium, and sulfur, are also found in egg whites. Eggs are a good source of the highest-quality protein on the face of the planet, as they contain all the amino acids we need in exactly the ratios we need.

MYTH: Brown eggs are better for us.
WHY WE THINK THAT: The color white represents "refined" while brown seems "earthy" and "unrefined." Advertisers know this and exploit it.

> *Eggs are a good source of the highest-quality protein on the face of the planet*

FACTS: Shell color has nothing to do with the nutritional value, quality, or flavor of the egg. Different breeds of hens simply lay different-colored eggs.

MYTH: We should only eat eggs with added omega-3.
WHY WE THINK THAT: If eggs contain omega-3 and are good for us, then eggs with even more omega-3 must be even better. It's "more is better" logic at work.

FACTS: The added omega-3 comes from what the chicken is fed, and the food value added is negligible compared to the cost. If you want to eat eggs with added omega-3 because those eggs taste better to you, that is fine.

MYTH: Organic eggs are better.
WHY WE THINK THAT: A lot of us think that "organic" means "better," thus conclude that it certainly can't hurt to eat organic eggs.

FACTS: Organic eggs come from healthy chickens fed pure foods and often raised under humane conditions. Many people believe healthier, more humanely treated chickens lay tastier eggs. Organic eggs do have slightly more beta-carotene and omega 3 fatty acids. This difference in nutrition is often not worth the difference in the cost. My family has eaten both conventional and organic eggs. We find that the organic eggs do taste slightly better, but nutritionally they are so close to conventional eggs, it is not worth the vast difference in price.

MYTH: Buy local eggs.

WHY WE THINK THAT: A lot of us believe if we buy organic and/or local, we are getting a better product. Usually we are right.

FACTS: If we buy locally, we certainly know where our eggs are coming from, and they may taste better. Nutritionally, they are close to the same as the conventional eggs sold in grocery stores. Buying local and/or organic eggs versus conventional eggs is an individual decision, and there is no right or wrong choice.

The Final Word on Eggs

Eggs are an excellent source of protein and they contain all the essential amino acids needed by the human body. When eggs are eaten with foods lower in protein, the egg protein provides amino acids that are in short supply in those other foods. One-eighth of the weight of the egg is protein, which is found in both the yolk and the white. Although protein is more concentrated around the outside of the yolk, most of the protein is in the white. When evaluating other types of protein, egg protein is the standard against which all other foods are assessed because it is a 100% complete protein and thus has the highest biological value.

When evaluating other types of protein, egg protein is the standard against which all other foods are assessed.

Eggs contain all the vitamins, except vitamin C, and are a good source of all the B vitamins and all the fat-soluble vitamins (A, D, K, and E). Eggs contain most of the minerals that the human body requires for health: iodine (required to make thyroid hormones), and phosphorus (required for bone health), zinc (required for wound healing, growth, and fighting infection), selenium (an important antioxidant), calcium (required for bone growth and nerve function), and iron (the vital ingredient in red blood cells).

The fat in an egg is found almost entirely in the yolk, with very little in the white. Overall, an egg is 11.2% fat. Fat in eggs is mostly monounsaturated, with some saturated fat and a small amount of polyunsaturated fat. In other words, the majority of the fat contained in an egg is monounsaturated, "good" fat. Cholesterol and lecithin are fat-like substances that are found in egg yolks, and are essential for the structure and function of all cells in the body. Cholesterol helps to maintain the flexibility and permeability of cell membranes, and is a raw material for the fatty lubricants that helps keep the skin supple. Cholesterol is essential for the production of sex hormones and the essential metabolic hormone, cortisol, as well as vitamin D, and bile salts. Lecithin is involved in general lipid transportation in the blood and in the metabolism of cholesterol. The old saying about the apple should be changed to "an egg a day keeps the doctor away."

> *The old saying about the apple should be changed to "an egg a day keeps the doctor away."*

MYTH: To lower blood cholesterol, avoid seafood and shellfish.

WHY WE THINK THAT: We have been led to believe that eating foods containing cholesterol will increase our cholesterol levels. Shellfish are generally thought to contain fairly high levels of cholesterol.

THE FACTS: The dietary cholesterol found in seafood, such as shellfish and other meats, has little effect on blood cholesterol in most people. Shrimp, lobster, crab, and scallops may be high in dietary cholesterol, but are also high in omega-3.

What to take away

- Cholesterol, in its unoxidized form, is a necessary fat that is made by the liver, even when not contained in the diet.
- Cholesterol is used by our bodies to make our hormones.
- Physically active people use more cholesterol.
- High cholesterol levels do not come from the cholesterol in your diet. High cholesterol levels result from interference with your body's use of cholesterol.
- Cholesterol ratios are a better indicator than total cholesterol level of how healthy we are.
- Exercise is the way to improve your cholesterol levels and ratios.
- Blood sugar levels are a better predictor of heart disease.

15. HORMONES THAT AFFECT OUR EATING

Jack Sprat could eat no fat, his wife could eat no lean; and so,
betwixt them both, they licked the platter clean.
— Mother Goose

One of the most important concepts of weight management that we
need to understand is the effect that four hormones have on our metabolism. These hormones are insulin, glucagon, leptin, and ghrelin. The
human body's ability to survive on a limited food supply evolved
because of these four hormones. An excess of any of these hormones is
not conducive to good health and can cause excessive weight gain or
weight loss. Here in the U.S., the hormone that is usually the most troublesome is insulin, since excessive amounts of insulin in the body cause
weight gain. Once the weight is gained, the excessive amount of insulin
coursing through the body prevents the body from losing that weight.
Thus a vicious cycle is created. The macronutrient most responsible for
the production of excess insulin is carbohydrate, especially carbohydrates high in simple sugars and carbohydrates that are refined and
processed.

Insulin and glucagon are two
important hormonal regulators of
how the macronutrients are metabolized. Insulin signals that the body is
fed and promotes the storage of

> Here in the U.S., the hormone that
> is usually the most troublesome is
> insulin.

fuels in the form of sugar, both in the liver and in the muscle. Insulin
facilitates the entry of glucose into muscle and fat cells. If we consume
an abundance of fatty acids and glucose in the foods we eat, we store the
excess as fat.

Insulin causes the body to store energy and stops the use of fat as an
energy source to prepare us for long periods of time between meals.
Without insulin, humans would have starved. Insulin converts calories
into stored energy, typically as fat and glycogen. When insulin is secreted
in a balanced fashion, no problem is created for our metabolism. When

we eat excessive amounts of food, we secrete excessive amounts of insulin, which creates problems.

Glucagon allows the body to utilize energy by stimulating the breakdown of glycogen and inhibiting fat formation. Glucagon increases the release of stored glucose by the liver and stimulates the use of stored fat as a fuel. Glucagon mobilizes fat and glycogen from where it is stored as energy in our body so that we can do things like an Ironman race or, generations ago, forage all day to find food. Without glucagon our muscles could do no work.

It is important to keep a balance between these two hormones. Many of us here in the U.S. live our whole life in a high-insulin "fed state." Too little activity, three full meals a day and snacks add up to too many calories. Too much insulin is then secreted to drive too many calories into our cells, which store the excess food as fat. A look at the many of us who are overweight today, even young people, points to this hormonal imbalance: too much insulin and too little glucagon.

Since so many in our society live in an excessive insulin state, it is important to be aware of the dangers of excessive insulin. Every time we eat a meal or snack, our body secretes insulin into our bloodstream.

> *The more "simple sugars" and processed carbohydrates our food contains, the higher the insulin response.*

The more "simple sugars" and processed carbohydrates our food contains, the higher the insulin response. Processed carbohydrates cause a higher insulin response than fresh fruit or fresh vegetables. Protein and fats do not cause high insulin responses; on the contrary, protein tends to even out the insulin response. The way to reduce our insulin level is to reduce the frequency and/or the size of our meals and to balance the macronutrients in our meals by being selective about what we eat. That way the body is not living in a constant high-insulin "fed" state.

Here is what typically happens and how we wind up with excessive insulin: we eat a big, mostly carbohydrate breakfast made with processed starches and sugars, then go to work and sit in an inactive state for most of the day. We continue to ingest snacks, such as doughnuts, followed by a big lunch, often of fast food. Lunch is usually followed by a feeling of lethargy and then a snack or two in the afternoon. Then we come home to dinner or go out to dinner, followed by a late-night snack. This leaves our body with high levels of insulin from early morning all the way until bedtime. Throughout the day, we have consumed too many calories, many from highly processed sources, and we have expended very few calories. High levels of insulin, just like high levels of glucose in our blood, are associated with many lifestyle diseases, such as diabetes, heart disease, cancer, arthritis, and, of course, obesity.

Thus, insulin supports the storage of food energy while glucagon supports the use of stored energy. An excess of either leads to problems. Excess glucagon is rarely seen here in the U.S. except in some cases of anorexia. However, since we have an obesity epidemic, one does not have to look far to see the effects of excessive insulin.

If we eat three separate meals, each containing only one of the macronutrients, the protein meal would cause the least amount of weight gain because a large percentage of calories from protein are *Of all the macronutrients, protein has the highest thermic effect.* burned off in the digestion process in what is called the thermic effect. Of all the macronutrients, protein has the highest thermic effect, burning off during digestion approximately 25% of the calories consumed as protein. In comparison, only 15% of the calories from carbohydrates are burned off during digestion, and fat has virtually no thermic effect whatsoever. Thus, all other things being equal, a high-protein diet would be less likely to cause fat deposition than either a high-carb or high-fat diet.

Moreover, unlike carbs, protein doesn't stimulate a significant insulin response. Insulin is a storage hormone and, while its primary purpose is to lower blood sugar, it also is responsible for shuttling fat into adipocytes (fat cells). When carbohydrates are ingested, the pancreas secretes insulin to clear sugar from the bloodstream. Depending on the quantities and types of carbs consumed, insulin levels can fluctuate wildly, increasing the likelihood of fat storage. Since protein's effect on insulin secretion is negligible, protein's potential for increasing fat storage is low.

What's more, the consumption of protein tends to increase the production of glucagon, the hormone that opposes the effect of insulin. Since a primary function of glucagon is to signal the body to burn fat for fuel, fat loss rather than fat gain tends to be promoted by protein consumption.

The other two hormones that affect our metabolism are leptin and ghrelin. Leptin was discovered in 1995 and is an appetite-suppressing hormone produced in the fat cells.

Fat loss rather than fat gain tends to be promoted by protein consumption.

Ghrelin is an appetite-stimulating hormone and is secreted by glands in the stomach to signal that we are hungry. Before we start to eat, the levels of ghrelin are high, signaling our brain that we need to find food. Once we start to eat, those levels start to decrease.

When we eat, leptin, ghrelin's counterpart, sends a signal to the brain that tells us we are satisfied and full, and ideally we stop eating. Leptin is secreted by our fat stores. When a person is overweight, they become leptin-resistant. The signal that should go to the brain to signal "I'm full" becomes blocked. Ironically, the more fat a person has, the more leptin is produced, but the signal gets diverted and doesn't reach the brain. When the leptin signal doesn't get to our brain, more insulin is produced to compensate for the extra amount of food we eat because we don't know we are full. In turn, the increased insulin continues to suppress the release of glucagon.

Too much ghrelin causes us to feel hungry, to stop using calories, and, instead, to store them. Leptin and ghrelin become unbalanced when we lose sleep. In the U.S., the

These is a definite association between increased weight and a lack of a good night's sleep.

amount of sleep we get per night has decreased as obesity has increased. Epidemiological studies on short sleep duration (SSD) and obesity have been conducted in children and adults and show a definite association between increased weight and a lack of a good night's sleep.[47] The two hormones that control appetite, leptin and ghrelin, have been studied as part of SSD's mechanism for causing obesity. Low leptin and high ghrelin levels have been seen in sleep deprivation. The effect is an increase in appetite along with a lack of feeling full, which are both linked to obesity. When we sleep, leptin tells the brain we are full and satisfied, so we stay asleep. However, when we have trouble sleeping, the hormone ghrelin is secreted and tells us we are hungry and that we need to store the calories we take in. On the other hand, leptin is suppressed, so we stay in a state of hunger without getting the signal that we are satisfied and full.

Here is what happens when these hormones are out of balance. With too much ghrelin in our system, we are stimulated to constantly feel hungry. This means we also will have too much insulin coursing through our bodies, and at the same time we won't have enough leptin to signal that we are full, so we will continue to eat. Glucagon will also be suppressed at the same time, so we will not be able to access our fat stores for fuel.

People who suffer from anorexia have unbalanced hormones, but in the opposite way. Anorexics have too much leptin in their systems, causing them to feel full even when they need to eat. At the same time, their ghrelin and insulin are suppressed, and glucagon is increased.

> *Anorexics have too much leptin in their systems, causing them to feel full even when they need to eat.*

The process of how our hormones work is a lot more complicated than I have described here, but this basic explanation will hopefully help you understand how your body works and the importance of hormonal balance.

What to take away

- Hormones are very important for how our bodies work, and they need to be kept in balance.
- Leptin gives us the "I'm full" signal, and ghrelin tells us "I'm hungry."
- Insulin promotes fat storage, and glucagon promotes fat usage.
- Hormones are more powerful than any drug.

16. HIGH-PROTEIN AND LOW-CARBOHYDRATE DIETS

I feel about airplanes the way I feel about diets. It seems to me they are wonderful things for other people to go on.
— Jean Kerr

Mosquitoes remind us that we are not as high up on the food chain as we think.
— Tom Wilson

As a fitness instructor, I'm often asked about high-protein and low-carbohydrate diets. Those questioning me think they know what constitutes a low- or high-protein diet, but with each person it is always something different. Time and again I hear speakers and writers, especially in the mass media, misrepresent experts, such as Dr. Barry Sears, who created the Zone Diet, as promoting a "high-protein" diet that is devoid of carbohydrates.[48] Sears recommends a dietary distribution of about 40% carbohydrates, 30% protein, and 30% fat. Is that a "high-protein" diet? If you're a government agency or a traditionally trained dietitian who believes we should consume only 12% of our calories from protein, then it is. I think of the Zone Diet as a "protein-adequate" diet. In fact, the main source of nutrition in the Zone Diet is carbohydrates.

The dietary guidelines recommended by Sears and other authors promoting low-carbohydrate diets do not really constitute a "low-carb diet," although the American Dietetic Association (ADA) might disagree. To the ADA, anything less than 55-60%, and sometimes even more, of our daily calories from carbohydrates is too low. Personally, I think this is unbalanced. I'll tell you why in this chapter.

Carbohydrates are paradoxical in that we need them but we don't have to directly consume them.

Carbohydrates are paradoxical in that we need them but we don't have to directly consume them. Let's consider the Eskimos and the

Masai, two human groups who do not directly consume carbohydrates. Before Eskimos met Europeans, they ate virtually no carbohydrates. What crops did they grow? What orchards did they tend on their white, frozen, ice shelf? They subsisted on fish, whales, seals, and a few land animals. The Eskimos still do not have fields or orchards. The Masai in Africa subsist on a diet of cow's blood mixed with cow's milk. Although tubers, berries, and grains are available, the Masai don't eat these, yet they are tall, slim, and healthy people. Ernest Shackelton's crew survived months stranded in the Antarctic on nothing but dog meat until it ran out and then on whale blubber.

How did the Eskimos, the Masai, and Shackelton's men get the vitamins and minerals that we get from carbohydrates? First of all, the

> *Pure carbohydrate has no known unique use in the human body.*

human body actually requires fats and proteins for various metabolic and physiological functions. Pure carbohydrate has no known unique use in the human body as the body can convert either fats or proteins as required into blood glucose, as it does with carbohydrate. Since these people we're considering eat their protein and fats raw, the vitamins and minerals from the carbohydrates the food animals consumed are still present in the blood, milk, skin, and muscle tissue. For instance, a serving of *muktuk* (raw skin with blubber) from the beluga whale contains the same amount of vitamin C as an orange. Once meat is heated, the nutrients from the carbohydrates that animal consumed are cooked and destroyed.

Unless you are one of the lucky people in the American populace whose metabolism operates flawlessly without disturbances in insulin metabolism or blood sugar levels, who does not struggle with a weight problem, who eats enough fiber in the form of whole and unrefined foods, who has no discernible food intolerances or sensitivities, who exercises daily, and who seems able to effortlessly process a highly grain-based diet, you're going to have a problem with the typical American high-carb, low-protein, low-fat diet.

In an attempt to banish fat from the American diet, we have replaced it with more carbs, processed sugars and starches than our Paleolithic digestive systems were ever designed to handle. Furthermore, those carbs are not the "good" kind that well-meaning nutritionists urge us to eat. They are processed, refined, and full of hidden sugars and bleached flours, devoid of nutrients, and loaded with calories. These foods may be low in fat, but they're making us sick and they're making us fat.

Over the last 40 years, during which the obesity epidemic has exploded, the only macronutrient amount that has not changed is the amount of protein we eat. What has changed is the amount of carbohy-

> *Our bodies need a specific amount of protein, and will continue to prompt us to eat until that amount is met.*

drates we eat, which are often found in processed foods that contain very little protein. Since our bodies need a specific amount of protein, and will continue to prompt us to eat until that amount is met, we end up overconsuming carbohydrates and fats found in protein-deficient processed foods.

The FDA dietary guidelines were designed for weight stability and health. There are people who will need more calories than are recommended, and some who will need less. There are people who will be able to eat more starches or fruit but that's what individualizing and customizing a plan is all about. The percentage of calories coming from carbohydrates in a higher protein diet is a bit less than the nutritional specialists believe we should be eating, but if the "official government-approved" version of what we should be eating worked well, we wouldn't have our current obesity epidemic!

Regardless of whose low-carb diet you try to follow, they all have a similar template. There are four basic phases to the diets. The initial phase is called the induction phase, which generally lasts two weeks and usually consists of lowering our carbohydrate intake to 20% of our total calorie intake. This is followed by a succession of phases where carbohydrates are slowly added back into the diet. Dietary problems are caused by how these diets are interpreted and followed. The initial phase is the one for people who are insulin-resistant and cannot process carbohydrates properly. By eating a substantially lower-carbohydrate, high-protein diet for two weeks, the body is potentially switched back to insulin sensitivity. Once the body is insulin-sensitive again, we can gradually add carbohydrates back into our diet until we reach our saturation level. The amount of carbohydrates each person can accommodate is different. The final phase is the maintenance phase, which generally breaks down to around 40% carbohydrate, 30% protein, and 30% fat.

The problem is that too often we stop reading the books at the chapter that explains the two-week phase and, since we tend to believe more is better, we assume that if two weeks of this works, four weeks

> *The problem is that too often we stop reading the books at the chapter that explains the two-week phase.*

will work better, and six weeks will be even better. Many people put themselves on a high-protein diet for a long period of time, and never get to the end of the book! Actually, the low-carbohydrate portion of the diet is meant to be the catalyst for an improved, balanced diet that includes a healthy representation of all of the macronutrients.

When an insulin-resistant person's body switches back to insulin sensitivity, they lose the water weight that was locked up by the excess sugar in their system. Many confuse this water loss with fat loss, which it is not. However, I don't think anyone who loses 15-20 pounds of water would want it back. As people continue on the diet in the correct fashion, they learn about healthy, nutritious food choices and what a reasonable portion size is. If we would take the time to really read the books, be they South Beach, Atkins latest edition, or Dr. Phil McGraw's diet book, we would see that each proposes a lifestyle change that incorporates exercise and education, not just a diet.

The same can be said for the high-carbohydrate diets, such as the one popularized by Dr. Ornish. Again, the final breakdown of the percentages of the macronutrients at the conclusion of those types of diets is around 40% carbs, 30% protein, and 30% fat. These diets support a change in lifestyle by eating healthy, nutritious foods in a balanced fashion, using reasonable portion sizes combined with more exercise. The rest is fluff, flash, and hype. Let's look at some more myths.

MYTH: Low-carbohydrate equals no-carbohydrate.
WHY WE THINK THAT: We hear media hype and gossip in the health clubs and among our friends that supports this belief.

THE FACTS: Many haven't read the high-protein, low-carbohydrate diet books thoroughly and end up believing what they have heard is "fact." The misconception is that a "low-carbohydrate" diet must be exceptionally low in carbohydrates or even eliminate carbohydrates. Not one low-carbohydrate diet advocates this. Even the Atkins induction phase, which is very low in carbohydrates, has some carbs and is only meant to last two weeks. According to the Atkins website, people who are not excessively overweight can skip the induction phase altogether.

Diet plans that recommend reducing carbs suggest that the carbohydrate level should be adjusted to the individual. Over the years, dieticians have been gradually lowering the range of recommended carbohydrates in the average diet.

> *Diet plans that recommend reducing carbs suggest that the carbohydrate level should be adjusted to the individual.*

They still continue to condemn reduced-carb diets, even though some of them now recommend the lower end of the new accepted range. Dr. Dean Edell, a prominent media physician, once stated that Dr. Barry Sears' Zone Diet, which contains 40% carbohydrate and is a low saturated-fat diet, "could be dangerous" because it is too low in carbohydrates. Yet the National Academy of Sciences now recommends that 45-65% of our diet be carbohydrate, depending upon the needs of the individual. This is not so different from the recommendations of the Zone Diet.

MYTH: Low-carbohydrate diets will cause weight gain.

WHY WE THINK THAT: If we want to lose weight, we have been encouraged to eat "rabbit" food.

THE FACTS: Research done by Stephen Simpson from the University of Sydney in Australia found that the body will demand food until its protein needs are met. If the need can be met with a serving of chicken, fish, meat, or eggs, fine. However, if the protein comes from sources of incomplete protein, such as bread, pasta, and rice, we will continue to eat until we have met our protein needs. Often this means overeating on high-carbohydrate foods in an effort to obtain enough protein.

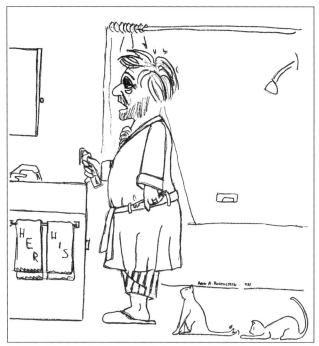

So, what new diet will I try today?

MYTH: Low-carb diets discourage eating vegetables and fruit.

WHY WE BELIEVE THAT: Many have not read the diet books first-hand and are going by what the "experts" say. By the way, the "experts" often haven't read the books either!

THE FACTS: Because vegetables and fruits are mainly carbohydrate, we believe that they are not allowed by low-carb diets when, in fact, the opposite is true. Non-starchy vegetables replace grains in the first phase of most of these diets because non-starchy vegetables don't raise our blood sugar level as fast or as high as grains do. People who follow a low-carb way of eating almost always eat more green vegetables than the general population. For the most part, green vegetables and low-glycemic fruits are the only carbohydrates eaten when following the first part of a low-carb diet. Later on, other colorful vegetables and fruits are added into the diet until a balance of about 40% carbohydrates, 30% protein, and 30% fat is achieved.

Research from the University of Washington showed that simply increasing the amount of protein in our diet helps us lose weight even if we don't shun carbohydrates one bit. Protein makes up 15% of most Americans' daily caloric intake, while fat accounts for 35% and carbohydrates for 50%. In the study, subjects bumped up their protein intake to 30% and reduced their fat intake to 20%. Within three months, they were eleven pounds lighter on average, even though half of the calories they ate still came from carbohydrates. The group also reported feeling satisfied with less food. In other words, they lost weight because they consumed fewer calories.[49] Extra protein, it turns out, sends "I'm full!" messages to the brain.

Protein's benefits go well beyond waistline trimming. The brain and its long spidery neurons are essentially made of fat, but the

Extra protein sends "I'm full!" messages to the brain.

neurons communicate with each other via proteins. The hormones and enzymes that cause chemical changes and control all body processes are also made of proteins. Carbohydrates, while essential as the brain's main source of fuel, can make us feel tired because they increase the brain's level of the amino acid, tryptophan. This, in turn, spurs production of the calming neurotransmitter, serotonin. Protein, on the other hand, prompts the brain to manufacture norepinephrine and dopamine, chemical messengers that promote alertness and activity.

MYTH: Low-carb diets have inadequate fiber.

WHY WE THINK THAT: Since fiber is found in foods containing carbohydrates, we think that a low-carbohydrate diet must be low in fiber. Since we believe "low-carb equals no-carb," how can there be any fiber? *Notice how one myth will perpetrate another!*

THE FACTS: Since fiber remains undigested and thus lessens the impact of other carbohydrates on blood sugar, high-fiber carbohydrates are recommended when following a low-carbohydrate diet. Lots of low-carbohydrate foods are high in fiber. In diets that encourage carbohydrate counting, fiber reduces the insulin-raising effect of the carbohydrates. Here is a list of the high-fiber carbohydrates that are encouraged in the induction phase of a low-carbohydrate diet:

Table 8: Some high-fiber carbohydrates

• Sprouts (bean, alfalfa, etc.)	• Peppers (green bell, red bell, jalapeno peppers)
• Greens: lettuces, spinach, chard, collards, mustard greens, kale, radicchio, endive, leeks, bok choy & celery	• Summer squash
	• Zucchini
	• Scallions or green onions, onions
• Herbs: parsley, cilantro, basil, rosemary, thyme, etc.	• Bamboo shoots
• Radishes	• Brussels sprouts
• Sea Vegetables (nori, etc)	• Snow peas (pods)
• Cabbage (or sauerkraut)	• Tomatoes
• Mushrooms	• Eggplant
• Jicama	• Tomatillos
• Avocado	• Artichokes
• Cucumbers (or pickles without added sugar)	• Fennel
	• Okra
• Asparagus	• Spaghetti squash
• Green beans and wax beans	• Celery root (celeriac)
• Broccoli	• Carrots
• Cauliflower	• Turnip
	• Water chestnuts
	• Pumpkin

MYTH: People eating low-carb diets are going to have heart disease.

WHY WE THINK THAT: We believe what the pundits say.

THE FACTS: In study after study, blood pressure, cholesterol, triglycerides, and other markers for increased risk of heart disease declined rather than increased on low-carb diets. In one large, long-term study, even low-carb diets with a lot of animal fat and protein did not raise the risk of heart disease.

MYTH: Low-carb diets will damage the kidneys.

WHY WE BELIEVE THAT: We believe that a high-protein diet means eating nothing but protein or excessive amounts of protein. Since protein is harder to digest than carbohydrates or fats, we assume that the excessive amounts of protein consumed in these diets will damage our kidneys.

THE FACTS: This has never been shown to be the case and, in fact, a low-carb diet is often not any higher in protein than the latest recommended dietary levels. The reduced amount of carbohydrates,

There is no evidence that a diet high in protein has any detrimental effects on those with normal kidney function.

mostly in the form of grains and sugar, reduces the total intake of calories and leads to weight loss. There is no evidence that a diet high in protein has any detrimental effects on those with normal kidney function. Consider that over the past century, millions of athletes have consumed large quantities of protein without incident. Surely, if high-protein diets caused kidney disease, these athletes would all be on dialysis by now! Not one peer-reviewed journal has documented any kidney abnormalities due to an increased intake of protein in healthy, active adults.

MYTH: Low-carb diets will "suck the calcium out of your bones."

WHY WE BELIEVE THIS: This is based on the myth that low-carb diets are always very high in protein. Some believe that people on higher protein diets tend to have more calcium in their urine.

THE FACTS: Rather than cause bone loss, protein actually protects our bones. Protein is used to replenish and rebuild our body's cells. Again, these diets don't advocate an overabundance of protein, they advocate controlling our insulin levels to prevent fat storage. By the time we are at the maintenance stage of any of these diets, we are consuming only 30% of our food in the form of protein.

MYTH: Dr. Atkins "died of his own diet."

WHY WE BELIEVE THIS: When a rumor is repeated often enough, it becomes "fact."

THE FACTS: Dr. Robert Atkins, originator of the Atkins Diet, died from head injuries resulting from a fall. He was not overweight when he died, as has been rumored. He retained a lot of fluid in the hospital while in intensive care after his injury.

MYTH: High-protein diets are high in saturated fat.

WHY WE THINK THAT: Some of the earlier editions of Dr. Atkins' diet books, as well as *Dr. Carlton Frederick's Low-Carbohydrate Diet* and *the L-C Diet (the Low Carbohydrate Diet),* did not differentiate between the different types of fats. That was almost 40 years ago! However, these books were once vilified by other dieticians, and the myth has remained.

THE FACTS: It is important to realize that certain fats, specifically the omega fatty acids, are actually necessary to our health and well-being because they aid in the absorption of fat-soluble vitamins

> *It is important to realize that certain fats, specifically the omega fatty acids, are actually necessary to our health and well-being.*

and facilitate the production of cell membranes, various hormones, and prostaglandins. These essential fats cannot be manufactured by the body and must be obtained from our food. Cold-water fish, such as salmon, mackerel, and trout, tofu, and peanut butter are protein-based foods that are also terrific sources of essential fats. Their consumption has been shown to have a positive impact on cardiovascular health and to reduce the risk of several types of cancers. The new low-carbohydrate diet books make a distinction between the different types of proteins and fats. Atkins' latest edition is a completely different book than the first one that came out in 1972.

What to take away

- Low-carb diets can be nutritious.
- Low-carb diets include high-quality carbohydrates.
- Lower-carb diets still have more carbohydrates than protein: 40% carbs, 30% protein, and 30% fat.
- The induction phase of a low-carb diet is only for those who are insulin-resistant.
- Low-carb and high-carb diets are balanced pretty much the same way.
- Losing weight is still all about total calories and increased activity.

17. SUGAR AND SUGAR SUBSTITUTES

I really don't think I need buns of steel. I'd be happy with buns of cinnamon.

— Ellen DeGeneres

Why have a separate chapter about sugar and not one about not flour, butter, or steak? Because sugar is found in practically everything, not just cookies, cakes, and candy. Sugar is one of the cheapest, most abundant, and most commonly used foods. It is found alone or as a hidden additive in other foods, such as seasoned salts, salad dressings, lunchmeats, beef jerky, and rotisserie chicken. These are foods that by definition should not have sugar and should not be sweet. Therefore, of all the foods, sugar is the easiest to consume in excess, often without knowing it's there.

The average person consumes 128 pounds of sugar a year, which is 34 teaspoons a day. The consequences are tooth decay and obesity. Sugar is a refined food that has been

> *Of all the foods, sugar is the easiest to consume in excess, often without knowing it's there.*

stripped of all vitamins, minerals, fiber, and water, and thus provides calories without nutrition. These terms may refer to sugar in a food product: *syrup*, *honey*, *molasses*, *corn sweeteners*, words ending in -ose, such as *dextrose*, *sucrose*, *lactose*, *maltose*, and the most common, *high-fructose corn syrup* or *HFCS*.

Even though sugar doesn't have nutritional value, if it is used for its intended purpose and not in excess, it can make eating a real pleasure. Sugar used as a flavoring makes otherwise unpalatable, bitter food enjoyable and edible. A great example is cocoa. Unrefined cocoa is extremely bitter, but add a little sugar and it becomes a wonderful treat. Sugar used sparingly as a flavor enhancer or eaten in a confection as a treat is not bad, so sugar should not be vilified. Eating it in excess is what causes problems. Now let's dispel some the myths surrounding sugar.

MYTH: Sugar causes diabetes.
WHY WE THINK THAT: Since we all associate diabetes with sugar intake and control, it is easy to assume sugar is the primary cause.

THE FACTS: This is probably the most common misconception about diabetes and about sugar. If you have diabetes, you need to watch your sugar and carbohydrate intake, with the help of a physician and a registered dietitian, to properly manage your blood sugar level. However, if you do not have diabetes, sugar intake will not cause diabetes. Instead, the main risk factors for acquiring the most common kind of diabetes, type II, are excess weight, a sedentary lifestyle, and a diet that is too high in overall calories.

A study published in *Diabetes Care* (April 2003)[50] re-confirmed that sugar does not cause diabetes.

If you do not have diabetes, sugar intake will not cause diabetes.

In this study, researchers analyzed data from nearly 39,000 middle-aged women based on a 131-item food questionnaire. Six years later, 918 women had developed type II diabetes. While many of the women reported diets high in sweets and carbohydrates, only a small percentage developed diabetes. Researchers found no definitive connection between sugar intake and the risk of developing type II diabetes. That doesn't mean we can eat all the sugar we want. Although consuming lots of sugar does not cause diabetes, consuming excessive calories from any source may. Because sugar is so easy to come by and is found in so many of our foods, excess caloric intake often is due to eating excess sugars. Excess caloric intake results in becoming overweight which is the main risk factor for diabetes.

The bottom line: Although excessive sugar intake is not the direct cause of type II diabetes, it can cause us to become overweight, which is one of the major risk factors. Maintaining a healthy weight and following a healthy lifestyle, including regular physical activity and a sensible diet, will help prevent type II diabetes.

MYTH: Type II diabetes can be prevented by eating foods low on the glycemic index.
WHY WE THINK THAT: Since we believe the previous myth, we use the glycemic index to find foods that are low in sugar.

THE FACTS: High sugar intake is not what causes diabetes; the disease is caused by the body's resistance to insulin. Foods with a high glycemic index can cause glucose levels to spike, pushing the body to become more resistant to insulin, but insulin resistance just indicates the possible presence of diabetes, not the root cause.

MYTH: High-fructose corn syrup (HFCS) is more fattening than regular sugar.

WHY WE THINK THAT: The media is full of negative statements about HFCS. We know that HFCS is bad, just not exactly why or how.

THE FACTS: This myth came from a 1968 study where rats were fed large amounts of fructose and developed high levels of fat in their bloodstreams.[51] Then, in 2002,

> Both HFCS and sucrose (table sugar) contain similar amounts of fructose.

researchers at the University of California at Davis published a paper noting that Americans' increasing consumption of fructose, including fructose found in HFCS, paralleled our skyrocketing rates of obesity. Both HFCS and sucrose (table sugar) contain similar amounts of fructose.[52] For example, the two most commonly used types of HFCS are HFCS-42 and HFCS-55, which are 42% and 55% fructose, respectively. Sucrose is almost chemically identical, containing 50% fructose. The truth is that the percentages of fructose in these two types of sugars, HFCS and table sugar, are so close that there's no evidence to show that one is significantly worse than the other. Both will cause weight gain when consumed in excess. HFCS and regular table sugar are empty-calorie carbohydrates that should be consumed in limited amounts by keeping soft drinks, sweetened fruit juices, and prepackaged desserts to a minimum in our diet.

One reason HFCS is thought to be more fattening is because it is commonly found in nutrient-deficient, calorie-dense foods. Table sugar is more often used sparingly to sweeten half a grapefruit or in the preparation of whole-food recipes, thus retaining a higher status. HFCS has a bad reputation because it's found in junk food and soda pop which, when consumed excessively, are known to cause weight problems. There appears to be evidence that HFCS blocks the feeling of being satisfied, so we may consume larger portions of foods products sweetened with HFCS than with regular sugar.

HFCS is found in a wide range of foods, such as ketchup, BBQ sauce, salad dressings, seasoned salts, cereals, boxed dinners, baked goods, and prepared lunchmeats. It's not that HFCS is worse than sugar; the problem is that HFCS is found in almost everything we eat. In addition, many of those foods are not in their whole, natural state. The result is more sugar in our diets than we need or can handle, thus making us overweight, which puts us at risk to become diabetic.

HFCS may block the feeling of being satisfied.

MYTH: Sugary foods make kids hyperactive.

WHY WE THINK THAT: Kids naturally are active, and we often see them being active while eating or drinking a sweet treat, so we put the two together and assume that sugar makes them hyper. After a party or after coming in from collecting Halloween candy, children seem overly active and excited.

THE FACTS: Studies have consistently found no relationship between sugar and hyperactivity. Children become rowdy and uncontrollable due to lack of sleep, poor diets, inadequate iron in their diet, excessive television or computer games, too much caffeine, too little physical activity, general excitement, such as a birthday party or Halloween activities, and a lack of discipline or parental supervision.

Studies have consistently found no relationship between sugar and hyperactivity.

Try feeding children healthy snacks that give them energy and nutrients, such as plain popcorn, whole fruits and vegetables, or whole-wheat crackers with cheese, peanut butter, soy butter, or bean dip. If they refuse these items, they are not hungry, so don't push food. If a child claims to be thirsty, offer them water. If that child refuses water but asks for soda, they are not thirsty. People who are hungry and thirsty take what is offered. Taking a gentle yet firm hand in monitoring what children do and what they consume will go a long way towards keeping them under control and not hyperactive.

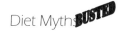

MYTH: Brown sugar is better than white sugar.

WHY WE THINK THAT: We have been conditioned to equate the color brown with "unrefined" and "healthy" and the color white with "refined" and "unhealthy," so brown sugar must be healthier and better.

THE FACTS: The brown sugar sold in grocery stores is really white, granulated sugar mixed with a minute amount of molasses so it will look brown. Brown sugar contains miniscule amounts of minerals, so the difference in mineral content between brown sugar and white sugar is insignificant. We can become overweight or obese on either of these sugars if we eat too much.

The brown sugar sold in grocery stores is really white...

MYTH: Honey is a better choice than sugar.

WHY WE THINK THAT: Since honey can be consumed in its raw state, we think it is healthier than white sugar, which is in a refined state.

THE FACTS: Honey and sugar are chemically similar and have close to the same calorie content but they taste different. Both honey and sugar contain four calories per gram. Sugar is made of glucose and fructose and has 49 calories per tablespoon. Honey is made of glucose, fructose, and a small amount of galactose and has 64 calories per tablespoon. Since honey is sweeter than sugar, we can use less to achieve the same desired sweetness as sugar. Children under one year of age should not be fed honey due to possible reactions to the different pollens bees use in making the honey. Some people may prefer honey to sugar because of its distinctive flavor.

MYTH: You should never eat cookies, candy, or ice cream.

WHY WE THINK THAT: We tend to be a society of extremes. Everything is all or nothing. If we are going to eat healthy, we can't deviate one bit!

THE FACTS: Everyone needs a treat now and then. Avoiding fun foods will bring on a desire to satisfy cravings and drive us to overindulge in these foods. Remember to eat these kinds of food sparingly, only as special treats.

MYTH: Since preschoolers lose their teeth, cavities from sweets don't matter.

WHY WE THINK THAT: Baby teeth are disposable, so why worry?

THE FACTS: Cavities can cause baby teeth to rot and fall out, which affects the placement of a child's permanent teeth. Baby teeth are more prone to cavities because their enamel is thinner. Even though they are stored up in the gum tissue, children's permanent teeth begin to harden as early as the first year of life, so good oral hygiene and a healthy diet are essential for the development of healthy permanent teeth. To prevent cavities, never allow a child to sleep with a bottle of juice or milk, brush your child's teeth after meals, have your child drink water after eating sweets if they can't brush right away, avoid frequent sweet snacks, use fluoride toothpaste, and visit the dentist regularly.

MYTH: Eating sugar, such as honey, candy bars, or marshmallows, will boost our energy levels when we feel low.

WHY WE THINK THAT: When we are hungry, our serotonin levels are low, so we feel tired and crave sweets and carbohydrates. Once refueled, we feel that resurgence of energy.

THE FACTS: Instead, the opposite will happen. A sugar snack is not nutritious and will negatively impact our workout or other activities by impeding our performance.

> *A sugar snack is not nutritious and will negatively impact our workout or other activities.*

The energy provided in a sugar snack will be used quickly, giving the illusion of more energy, but the false high will vanish quickly, leaving us feeling empty and tired.

Typically we are unaware of just how much sugar we eat throughout the day. Just 100 grams of sugar impairs our immune system and reduces our body's ability to capture and destroy bacteria.[53] These effects start 30 minutes after ingestion of sugar and can last for over five hours. Continuously eating sugar breaks down our immune barriers. It is easy to consume 100 grams of sugar if we are not careful. Just 10 gumdrops, or even healthy meals of oatmeal with raisins, a banana, and fruit juice, contain over 100 grams of sugar. Sugar is present in so many of our

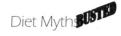
foods that we can easily overdo sugar consumption every day, year after year, pound after pound.

MYTH: Sweets are a good source of vitamins.

WHY WE THINK THAT: This is simply wishful thinking, especially if you are a child.

THE FACTS: Candy and other sweets contain large amounts of sugar but no vitamins, nutrients, or minerals. Consuming nothing but sugar is worse than trying to subsist on water alone.

> *Consuming nothing but sugar is worse than trying to subsist on water alone.*

We can live only three days without water and a few more days on food without water, since food contains moisture, but we can live up to fifteen days with no food as long as we have water. In 1793 an English ship carrying a sugar cargo was shipwrecked and five sailors were marooned for nine days. They couldn't drink the ocean water and had only sweet rum and sugar to sustain them. By the time they were rescued nine days later, they were severely malnourished, dehydrated, and close to death, despite the fact that all that rum and sugar contained lots of calories.

Sir Fredrick Banting, the codiscoverer of the hormone insulin, noticed in 1929 in Panama that diabetes was common among the sugar plantation owners who consumed refined sugar. Among the plantation workers, diabetes was unknown because the workers had access to only the raw sugar cane stalks, which they chewed raw.[54] We can guess that other effects, such as obesity and amount of exercise, were also involved.

Breaking down sugar requires the assistance of other nutrients. Excess sugar causes the body to become depleted of calcium, sodium, potassium, and magnesium, plus sugar attacks the immune system. The depletion of calcium causes the onset of osteoporosis.

The bottom line: Sugar is a pleasant-tasting additive that can make foods taste better. Used sparingly and responsibly, it is not a problem. Eating excessive amounts of sugar in any form causes cavities and weight gain and impairs our immune system, leading to the onset of various inflammatory diseases, such as heart disease, arthritis, diabetes, and cancer.

MYTH: Artificial sweeteners help us lose weight.

WHY WE THINK THAT: Since we aren't consuming calories from sugar, we have reduced our overall calorie intake.

THE FACTS: Yes and no. When we truly use artificial sweeteners as replacements for sugar, watch our calorie intake, and exercise, we are able to sustain a healthy weight. However, many of us use the sweeteners as a substitute for sugar, and then believe that we can consume more calories from other sources since we have fewer calories in our drinks or food as if to make up the difference. How many times have we overheard someone at a fast-food outlet order a super-sized meal along with a diet drink?

On a more serious note, artificial sweeteners seem to alter our metabolism and our brain chemistry. When we taste something sweet, our bodies prepare for the expected

Artificial sweeteners seem to alter our metabolism and our brain chemistry.

sugar calories, but when we use artificial sweeteners, those calories don't arrive. This confuses our bodies, and we continue to eat more to achieve the fulfillment of the expected calories. In a Purdue University study, rats fed artificial sweeteners experienced this physiological calorie expectation, and this drove them to overeat.

MYTH: Artificial sweeteners are unhealthy.

WHY WE THINK THAT: We think anything artificial is fake and therefore not as good as the real thing.

THE FACTS: A lot of the time this is true. Saccharin was banned in 1977 after studies showed it was linked to bladder cancer. However, only one study out of many showed a weak link between bladder cancer and the consumption of six or more servings a day of diet soda containing saccharin. In 2000 the National Toxicology Program removed saccharin from their list of carcinogens.

At the moment, there is no credible evidence that aspartame causes seizures, multiple sclerosis, Alzheimer's dementia, lupus, or allergic reactions. The connection between aspartame and cancer is less clear. In two different European studies in 2005 and 2007, rats fed aspartame in doses at or below the level considered safe in humans had increased risks of lymphoma, leukemia, and breast cancer. Since aspartame contains the amino acid phenylalanine, people with phenylketonuria (PKU), a sensitivity to phenylalanine, should avoid aspartame, as should women who are pregnant since there is no way to know if the fetus has PKU.

People who are diabetic need to avoid the sweeteners Estee and Sweet Simplicity because they contain fructose as a substitute for sugar and fructose will spike diabetics' insulin, just as table sugar does. Fructose also increases the levels of blood lipids (fats) which increases LDL (bad) cholesterol. The American Diabetes Association now recommends avoiding fructose but says diabetics may use table sugar in very limited amounts.

> *People who are diabetic need to avoid the sweeteners Estee and Sweet Simplicity.*

Stevia, an all-natural product from Peru, is an herbal sweetener, and does not require approval from the FDA. Stevia does not spike a person's insulin and is free of calories. Its flavor is stronger and sweeter than table sugar, so only a little is necessary. It makes a good substitute for sugar to sweeten grapefruit, cereal, or a beverage, but for cooking your favorite recipe from scratch, table sugar is best.

MYTH: Sugar-free foods don't have calories.

WHY WE THINK THAT: Any time we see the word "free" in association with food, we assume "zero calories."

THE FACTS: "Sugar-free" means there are no calories from sugar in the food but there are still calories from all of the other ingredients. This gives us a false sense of security, so we eat even more of the sugar-free item. Often, sugar-free foods not only don't have sugar, they also don't have adequate vitamins and minerals. Some research suggests that consuming too much artificial sweetener disrupts the body's ability to register calories, so the body doesn't feel full and therefore we continue to eat in an effort to achieve that full feeling. Of course, this leads to weight gain not weight loss.

The bottom line: Use both sugar and artificial sweeteners in moderation. Although sugar has no nutritional value, it is a real food, and

> *Use both sugar and artificial sweeteners in moderation.*

adds a pleasant flavor to many foods. If you must use artificial sweeteners, do so in moderation. When you want something sweet, try to consume ripe fruits when possible. They are free of added sugar, full of vitamins and nutrients, and taste great!

Calorie-loaded drink to avoid: Deemed the "Worst Drink in America" by Men's Health Magazine,[55] Cold Stone Creamery PB&C Shake. The 24-ounce "Gotta Have It" size packs 2,030 calories with 131 grams of fat (68 grams saturated and 2.5 grams trans fat) and 153 grams of sugars. This blended peanut-butter-cup concoction makes it possible to spend 10 minutes slurping down a drink that will take four hours of running on a treadmill to burn off. Baskin-Robins cut down on the calories in its drinks in the past couple of years, but ice cream-based drinks, regardless of who makes them, still are packed (and overpacked) with calories.

What to take away

- Sugar is not evil, but it should be used sparingly, as a treat, since it contains no nutrients or vitamins.
- Sugar does not cause hyperactivity or diabetes.
- Sugar is hidden in many processed and refined foods under many different names, so it is easy to consume too much. Read labels!

18. SALADS

Knock Knock. Who's there? Lettuce. Lettuce who? Lettuce in and you'll find out!

— Anonymous

Lettuce is a member of the daisy family Asteraceae. It is most often grown as a leaf vegetable. In many countries, it is eaten cold, raw, in salads, sandwiches, hamburgers, tacos, and in many other dishes. In some places, including China, lettuce is typically eaten cooked and use of the stem is as important as use of the leaf. Both the English name and the Latin name. *Lactuca sativa*, are ultimately derived from *lac*, the Latin word for milk referring to the plant's milky juice. The mild flavor of lettuce has been used over the centuries as a cooling counterbalance to other ingredients in a salad.

The lettuce plant has a short stem that looks like a small rose, but when it gradually blooms, the stem and branches lengthen; and produce many flower heads that look like those of dandelions, but smaller. This is referred to as bolting. When grown to eat, lettuce is harvested before it bolts. Some lettuces, especially iceberg, have been specifically bred to remove the bitter flavor from their leaves. These lettuces have high water content with very little nutrient value. The more bitter lettuces and the ones with pigmented leaves contain antioxidants.

> *The more bitter lettuces and the ones with pigmented leaves contain antioxidants.*

MYTH: It's just a low-calorie salad!

WHY WE THINK THAT: A salad is usually made with bulky foods that have little density, so it can't have many calories.

THE FACTS: At 490 calories and 41 grams of fat, there is nothing "just" about a Subway BMT salad with ranch dressing. That is more calories and fat than in a Burger King bacon cheeseburger, which contains 360 calories and 18 grams of fat. At Ruby Tuesday, the Carolina Chicken Salad packs 1,300 calories with 72 grams of fat. Add another

170

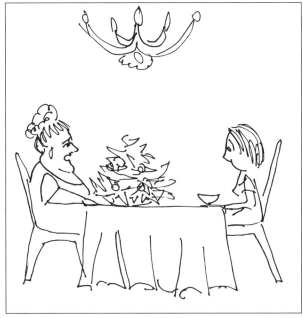

It's just a salad.

275 calories for the dressing! Many fast-food or restaurant salads contain low-quality, nutritionally poor lettuce and few nutritious vegetables. Most of these salads contain carrot shavings rather than whole pieces and often only one slice of a cucumber or tomato. What they do have in abundance is cream-style dressings that are often loaded with trans fat. At a salad buffet, we can pile our plates high with lettuce and more than the normal proportion of added condiments (calories), all topped with lots of dressing.

MYTH: Fat-free dressings are the healthiest.

WHY WE THINK THAT: If we believe fat is the root cause of our obesity problem, then using a dressing without fat would be healthier.

Fat-free dressings block our ability to absorb the antioxidants in salad greens and tomatoes.

THE FACTS: Not quite. We do save on calories when we take out the fat, but many such dressings replace the fat with sugar at more than two teaspoons per serving and offer zero nutrition. Fat-free dressings block our ability to absorb the antioxidants in salad greens and tomatoes, which are important compounds that reduce the risk of heart disease. In one study, people eating full-fat salad dressing absorbed twice the nutrients than those using reduced-fat dressing did. Fat-free dressing did not allow absorption of those good nutrients.

MYTH: Celery has negative calories.

WHY WE THINK THAT: This is an old wives' tale that just keeps on going.

THE FACTS: At six calories per stalk, celery is unquestionably a weight-friendly food. But the body doesn't expend more calories than those used to chew and digest it,

> *At six calories per stalk, celery is unquestionably a weight-friendly food.*

according to David Baer, PhD, a research physiologist at the USDA Beltsville Human Nutrition Research Center in Maryland. "No negative-calorie foods have been discovered yet," he says. If we really think about it, negative-calorie food is a silly idea since all living things need food to sustain them. A negative-calorie food goes against all basic physiological principles.

MYTH: Lettuce is lettuce.

WHY WE THINK THAT: How nutritious could a leaf be!?

THE FACTS: When it comes to nutrition and flavor, arugula and watercress are the superstars of the lettuce family because they are loaded with cancer-fighting compounds. In fact, a chemical in watercress has been shown to deactivate one of the cancer-causing toxins in tobacco smoke. Spinach is another great choice because it has an abundance of lutein, which is thought to protect against cancer and blindness. And baby versions of kale, mustard greens, and turnip greens are less sharp, tough, and bitter than the grown-up versions, and are outfitted with the same cancer-fighting nutrients. Dark-leaf, mild-tasting greens, such as romaine, red-leaf lettuce, and many mesclun mixes, don't have a wealth of phytonutrients, but do have respectable levels of beta-carotene. Light greens, such as iceberg and endive, are pretty much low in nutrition. These last two are the cheapest greens, and thus are what most restaurants and fast-food outlets use.

Along with superior choices of lettuce, colorful, all-vegetable salads offer other phytonutrients that aren't available in greens. For example, powerful antioxidants in purplish vegetables, such as eggplant, help reduce the risk of heart disease and improve brain function. Radishes offer cancer-fighting indoles, and red tomatoes contain lycopene, which reduces the risk of heart disease and cancer.

The bottom line: With salads, the more colorful the salad, the better it is nutritiously. Use colorful fruits and vegetables along with a variety of greens.

Myths: Garbanzo beans provide a meal's worth of protein.

WHY WE THINK THAT: We have been told over and over that beans contain protein.

THE FACTS: A ladleful of garbanzo beans, about ¼ cup, provides roughly four grams of protein, not nearly enough if that's the only protein you're having in that meal. We need 0.36 grams of protein per pound of body weight per day. For example, a 154-pound woman needs about 55 grams of protein daily. We get more protein by combining ¾ cup of beans containing 11 grams of protein with ¼ cup of chopped egg containing 4 grams of protein and ¼ cup of shredded cheese containing 7 grams of protein.

MYTH: If I add bacon to my salad, it will blow my diet, so I might as well have ordered a burger.

WHY WE THINK THAT: We think of bacon as being greasy and fattening, thus it is often called out as a food villain.

THE FACTS: Bacon won't ever win any trophies for being a health food but it's not as bad as it is made out to be. One slice is about 1½

Bacon is not as bad as it is made out to be.

tablespoons crumbled and has about the same amount of fat as 2 tablespoons of feta cheese, shredded cheddar cheese, or a tablespoon of sunflower seeds. We need to keep other fats, such as those found in croutons or creamy dressings, out of our salad because they contain trans fats as preservatives. Since conventional bacon is preserved with the known carcinogen, nitric oxide, feta cheese or sunflowers seeds would be a healthier choice. If you really like bacon, buy bacon that is locally butchered, so it doesn't need the preservatives.

MYTH: You can't get food poisoning from salad like you can from beef or chicken.

WHY WE THINK THAT: We tend to think that salads are fresh and that fresh food isn't spoiled.

THE FACTS: "Lettuce, sprouts, and tomatoes are some of the most common carriers of salmonella, toxic strains of E. coli, and other harmful microbes," said Christopher

> *Lettuce, sprouts, and tomatoes are some of the most common carriers of harmful microbes*

Braden, MD at the Centers for Disease Control in Atlanta. These germs get onto the food from the manure and contaminated water they're grown in. That is what was suspected in the E. coli/spinach fatalities in California in 2007.[56] The manure and contaminated water gets transferred to a dirty cutting board or knife, or from people touching the vegetables without washing their hands. There is not much we can do about it when we're eating out, but at home we can wash veggies under running water and keep our knives and cutting boards clean.

MYTH: Organic salad is healthier.

WHY WE THINK THAT: We believe anything organic must be better and healthier because it is more natural.

THE FACTS: When it comes to nutrients, freshness matters more than an "organic" designation. Every day, heat and light speed up the decline of picked vegetables,

> *When it comes to nutrients, freshness matters more than an "organic" designation.*

losing vitamin B, vitamin C, and other nutrients. A conventional head of lettuce that was picked yesterday and used today will deliver more nutrients than an organic head of lettuce that's been sitting on the store shelf for a week. Of course, there are reasons to choose organic, but a nutrient bonus isn't one of them unless you are going to use the item right away.

What to take away

- Lettuce and celery contain calories. There is no such thing as a negative-calorie food.
- For better nutrition, choose darker lettuce leaves.
- "Organic" is only better nutritionally when it is used as quickly as non-organic.

19. SEAFOOD

Why does Sea World have a seafood restaurant? I'm halfway through my fish burger and I realize: Oh my God! I could be eating a slow learner.
— Lynda Montgomery

In Mexico we have a word for Sushi: bait.
— Jose Simons

Seafood refers to any sea animal or plant that is served as food and eaten by humans. Seafood includes seawater animals, such as fish and shellfish. The harvesting of wild seafood is known as fishing and the cultivation and farming of seafood is known as aquaculture, mariculture, or in the case of fish, fish farming. Seafood is different from meat, although it is still animal and is excluded in a vegetarian diet. Seafood is an important source of protein in many diets around the world, especially in coastal areas.

Many myths and misconceptions about fish and seafood are handed down from generation to generation and grow with each telling until they become almost an inherent part of the culture in which they grew. Here are a few of the myths and misconceptions concerning fish and seafood that have come down through the years.

> Seafood refers to any sea animal or plant that is served as food and eaten by humans.

MYTH: Most fish contains mercury, so only eat fish occasionally.

WHY WE THINK THAT: The news media is good at sensationalizing the idea that fish is full of mercury.

THE FACTS: The way they print it, we might as well stick a fish in our mouth to take our temperature! Some fish from some areas contain mercury, but we need to keep the facts in perspective. The benefits of eating fish far outweigh the risks. A team of scientists at Harvard School of Public Health recently reported that the death rate from heart disease was 36% lower among people who ate fish twice a week compared with people who ate little or no fish. The study, which was published in the 18 October 2006 issue of the *Journal of the American Medical Association*, showed that overall mortality was 17% lower among the seafood eaters. Nearly all fish contains minute amounts of mercury. Among commercially available fish and shellfish in the United States, the most commonly eaten species, such as shrimp, canned light tuna, salmon, pollock, and catfish, contain almost no mercury and pose little risk.

Seafood is a rich source of the essential omega-3 fatty acids that have been shown to enhance brain and eye development in the fetus,

The benefits of eating fish far outweigh the risks.

promote a healthy pregnancy, aid thinking and learning during childhood, reduce the risk of heart disease and stroke, and slow mental decline as people age. It is because of all these health benefits that the U.S. Food and Drug Administration (FDA), the Environmental Protection Agency (EPA), the American Heart Association (AHA), and the 2005 U.S. Dietary Guidelines all recommend that Americans of ages two years and older eat two eight-ounce servings a week of a variety of fish and shellfish. Eat fish regularly because it's an important part of the diet and it's good for you!

MYTH: Pregnant and nursing women and children should stay away from fish because it contains mercury.

WHY WE THINK THAT: We tend to believe everything we read or hear, and then obsess and talk about it.

THE FACTS: Recent scientific research found that there are many health benefits from omega-3 fatty acids, including some specifically for women, infants, and young children. The FDA and EPA have issued special guidelines[57] for pregnant and nursing women, women who might become pregnant, and young children. Fish that are high in mercury and should be avoided are shark, swordfish, king mackerel, and tilefish (golden bass, golden snapper).

Fish that can be eaten in limited quantities by women who are/may be pregnant or nursing, and young children are

- canned light tuna
- sea bass
- Gulf Coast oysters
- eastern oysters
- marlin
- halibut
- channel catfish (wild)
- haddock
- mahi-mahi
- largemouth bass

- blue mussel
- cod
- pollock
- Gulf Coast blue crab
- pike
- Great Lakes salmon
- lake whitefish
- white croaker
- walleye

The FDA says that by women who are/may be pregnant or nursing, and young children can safely consume up to 12 ounces of fish that are extremely low in mercury, including:

- catfish (farmed)
- king crab
- scallops
- fish sticks
- flounder (summer)

- trout (farmed)
- Pacific salmon (wild)
- shrimp
- tilapia
- sardines

MYTH: All tuna is high in mercury and should be avoided.

WHY WE THINK THAT: The media's sound bites have us all nervous and scared about tuna.

THE FACTS: Actually, the amount of mercury in canned light tuna is tiny. Canned light tuna appears on the FDA's and EPA's

The amount of mercury in canned light tuna is tiny.

lists of commonly eaten fish that contains almost no mercury. Canned albacore (white) tuna and fresh tuna contain more mercury than light tuna, and the FDA and EPA recommend that pregnant and nursing women, women who might become pregnant, and young children limit their weekly consumption of canned albacore tuna and fresh tuna to no more than six ounces. Six ounces is about two average meals; young children should receive smaller portions than adults.

For the rest of the U.S. population, men of any age and women who do not plan to become pregnant or are past childbearing age, the health benefits of eating fish, including canned and fresh tuna, twice a week far outweigh the potential risks,

> *Government and public health groups encourage most people to eat more, not less, fish*

partly because current fish consumption levels are so low. Because only a small percentage of the general U.S. population currently eats fish at least two times per week, government and public health groups encourage most people to eat more, not less, fish and particularly recommend a variety of fish and shellfish. As one of the top ten most commonly consumed fish in the U.S., canned tuna is an excellent and affordable source of lean protein and certain essential vitamins and minerals. Moreover, the types of fats present in tuna are heart-healthy, help reduce the level of fats in the blood, and increase our level of "good" HDL cholesterol. Canned tuna is widely available packed in water for those who want to minimize calories from oil.

MYTH: If you eat fish, you are ingesting the same type of mercury found in a thermometer.

WHY WE THINK THAT: When we think of mercury, we are not thinking about the planet closest to the sun, we immediately think of the liquid metal inside a thermometer. That is because this is the only type of mercury many of us know about.

THE FACTS: Mercury exists in many different forms. That used in thermometers is elemental mercury. The type of mercury found in the ocean or in freshwater and consumed by fish is almost always bound to "organic," carbon-based compounds. The most common form in seafood is methylmercury.

MYTH: The levels of mercury in fish have gone up in recent years due to increased pollution and industrialization.

WHY WE THINK THAT: With more people in the world and more industrialization, it would make sense that there would be more mercury in our food supply.

THE FACTS: According to independent studies, the amount of mercury in fish, such as canned tuna, has not increased in the last 25 years. In fact, an EPA-funded Princeton University study

The amount of mercury in fish has not increased in the last 25 years.

compared mercury concentrations in yellow-fin tuna caught off the coast of Hawaii in 1998 with the amount of mercury in yellow-fin tuna caught in the same area in 1971.[58] That study found no increase in mercury levels. However, fresh tuna should still be eaten sparingly.

MYTH: Fatty acids in fish are bad for you and will lead to heart attacks.

WHY WE THINK THAT: It has been drummed into our heads that all fat and fatty acids are bad for us and lead to heart disease.

THE FACTS: The omega-3 fatty acids found in fish are especially important for building and maintaining brain tissue and the retina of the eye. They are most readily available from seafood, but tiny amounts can be obtained from plant-based omega-3 found in flax oil, walnuts, and canola oil. While generally not as effective as the omega-3 found in seafood, plant-based omega-3 is healthful. Omega-3 fatty acids help protect against cardiovascular disease because they reduce abnormal heart rhythms, lower triglyceride levels in the blood, slow the rate of plaque formation, and improve the health of our arteries. They can also reduce the risk of blood clots and stroke.

MYTH: All fish are good sources of omega-3.

WHY WE THINK THAT: The American Heart Association tells us to eat at least two servings of fish per week because fish is a good source of omega-3.

THE FACTS: Not all fish have high levels of omega-3. The best fish to consume for this heart-healthy fat are cold-water fish, such as salmon, fresh or canned rainbow trout, sardines, canned tuna, catfish, and anchovies. Wild-caught fish are usually a much better choice than farmed-raised fish. The fish-farming industry keeps its prices down by feeding their fish inexpensive food that can have an adverse effect on the nutritional quality of the fish. One popular farm-raised fish, tilapia, may actually harm our hearts due to its low levels of healthy omega-3 fatty acids and high levels of unhealthy omega-6 fatty acids. High levels of omega-6 have been connected to an increase in heart disease, arthritis, asthma, diabetes, and other inflammatory diseases.

While wild fish is generally superior, farmed trout and Atlantic salmon have relatively good concentrations of omega-3 fatty acids

> *The best fish to consume for this heart-healthy fat are cold-water fish.*

compared to omega-6 fatty acids. Farm-raised tilapia and catfish, on the other hand, have much higher ratios of omega-6 to omega-3. Wild fish can be bought fresh, frozen, or canned.

MYTH: Fish has a strong smell and tastes bad.

WHY WE THINK THAT: We all have had experiences with poorly prepared fish that lingers on in our memories.

THE FACTS: Fresh fish and shellfish have a mild taste and smell.

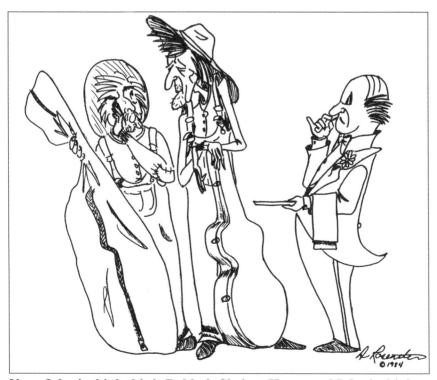

Vern, I don't think this is Bubba's Shrimp House and I don't think that fella there is Bubba.

The taste of different species, such as tuna, shrimp, and salmon, varies and there are many convenient ways to prepare fish to enhance the flavors we like best. Recipes for fish have come a long way since the days when our only choice was one brand of frozen fish sticks. Fish can be made into patties and used in tacos and chowders, fish steaks can be marinated and grilled, and fish can be baked instead of fried to make our meal lower in fat and calories. Canned tuna is one of the easiest types of fish to turn into snacks or quick, satisfying meals, yet it can be used for more sophisticated, gourmet meals. A wide variety of marinades and spices are available to tempt our palate and numerous recipes are easy to find.

MYTH: Oysters and other shellfish should not be eaten in months without an *R* in them.

WHY WE THINK THAT: This belief came about before adequate refrigeration. We all know that the months without an *r* in their names are the summer months of May, June, July, and August.

THE FACTS: As far as the United States is concerned, this is not true. Under commercial conditions for raising and harvesting, oysters and other shellfish are safe

> *Oysters and other shellfish are safe and good to eat any month of the year.*

and good to eat any month of the year. Certain European oysters that brood their young in months without an r are less palatable at that time of year, but this rule doesn't apply to U.S. oysters (which don't brood their young). In contradiction to the myth about eating shellfish only in *r* months, shellfish containing a paralytic poison are occasionally found along the Pacific Coast in *r* months. When this occurs, people are warned against gathering and eating those particular shellfish. The California Department of Health places a quarantine on the harvesting of mussels between May 1 and October 31. Along the Oregon Coast, people are warned by the news media against gathering and eating the mussels that cling to rocks that rim the beaches. The rule to follow is that any commercially available shellfish is non-toxic and safe to eat.

MYTH: Oysters are an aphrodisiac.

WHY WE THINK THAT: The idea of eating oysters for their aphrodisiac qualities has been around for a long time.

THE FACTS: Oysters contain considerable amounts of nature's building block, cholesterol, as well as being extremely rich in protein. An adequate amount of protein enhances our sexual abilities, although it is doubtful that this was common knowledge when the aphrodisiac myth was created.

MYTH: Shellfish that die before being cooked should not be eaten.

WHY WE THINK THAT: We have been warned not to eat clams, mussels, crabs, lobsters, and other shellfish unless they are alive when cooked.

THE FACTS: If this were really true, there would be a lot of empty space in the frozen food section at the grocery store! From the standpoint of flavor, this is a good suggestion, but shellfish don't become toxic when they die. When shellfish die, their digestive glands break down, releasing enzymes that begin digesting the flesh of the animal. Cooking the shellfish alive prevents this process from beginning. The reason you should only clean and cook live or fresh-frozen shellfish is that those that die before being cooked or frozen will have a decomposed flavor and odor. This goes back to the idea that fish taste bad and why.

Shellfish don't become toxic when they die.

MYTH: Seafood is brain food.

WHY WE THINK THAT: We have been told this and have read this so much that we assume it is true.

THE FACTS: The myth of fish as a brain food goes back to a 19th century scientist at Harvard University who discovered that phosphorus is abundant in the human brain and, from this fact, wrongly concluded that since fish is a good source of phosphorous a diet of fish should increase human intelligence.

MYTH: Mahi-mahi is dolphin meat.

WHY WE THINK THAT: This is both the name of a dolphin and a fish, but most of us only know it as a name for a dolphin.

THE FACTS: This myth probably originated because the fish mahi-mahi is also called "dolphin fish" or "dolphin." Mahi-mahi is really a fish caught in tropical waters and marketed throughout the world. The dolphin is a mammal protected by the 1972 Marine Mammal Protection Act and is not harvested or used for food in the United States.

MYTH: Frozen seafood is inferior to fresh seafood.

WHY WE THINK THAT: We assume anything fresh is superior to anything frozen or preserved in any way.

THE FACTS: There was some truth to this around the time the marketing of seafood went through a transitional period from simple refrigeration and icing methods to

Fresh-frozen seafood has exactly the same quality and flavor as it did when it was frozen.

more sophisticated freezing methods. The truth now is that fresh seafood is processed quickly after being harvested, and any surplus beyond immediate marketing demands is frozen by the "glaze" method, which literally coats the product with a layer of ice. This is an improvement over the old dry-freezing method, which itself was a viable way of handling a highly perishable product. Fresh-frozen seafood has exactly the same quality and flavor as it did when it was frozen.

What to take away

- Fresh-water fish, ocean fish, and other seafood are great sources of lean protein and omega-3.
- There is not enough mercury in commonly eaten fish to make it reasonable to eliminate fish from one's diet.
- Fish, just like any other food, should be eaten in moderation. Twice a week is a good rule of thumb.

20. ENERGY AND FOOD REPLACEMENT BARS AND ENERGY DRINKS

Health food may be good for the conscience but Oreos taste a hell of a lot better.

— Robert Redford

Americans buy energy bars, thinking they are a health food or a meal alternative. Energy bars are for people who think they need more immediate get-up and go and who look to an energy bar to give it to them. Energy bars promise to boost energy, and thus performance, in the form of an alternative meal or "power snack." The label says it'll supply us with vitamins and minerals and give us an energy high to rival a Caribou super-size latte. Boosted by these promises, Americans bought $1.8 billion worth of energy bars in 2002.

Many of these bars are loaded with sugar and fat, often trans fat so the bars can have a longer shelf life. They contain simple sugars and lack nutrition, so they can derail our diet and ultimately turn that energy surge into crash-and-burn.

When it comes to energy drinks, the same manufacturing claims apply. Raw fruits and vegetables contain a vast array of nutrients and most of us are not consuming enough fruits or vegetables. However, no single fruit or vegetable or any other food will ever be the solution for all of our ailments. What is best is a diverse diet.

The so-called super juices like goji, noni, mangosteen, and açai are pricey and come with a number of spurious and anecdotal health claims. The health claims of these juices are exaggerated, the products are overpriced, and the only way to purchase these items is through specialty distributors.

> *The so-called super juices like goji, noni, mangosteen, and açai are pricey and come with a number of spurious and anecdotal health claims.*

Here are the biggest myths about energy bars, according to nutritionists, as well as my own observations.

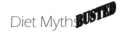

MYTH: Energy bars will boost the energy we need for a better workout.

WHY WE THINK THAT: Look at any ad for energy bars. They feature images of people running, leaping, biking, and being energetic. The bars claim to be meal replacements or supplements that are full of necessary vitamins and nutrients that will enhance our workouts.

THE FACTS: Experts say labeling a product an "energy food" is just a sly way of admitting it contains unnecessary calories. "It's not like you're going to be able to leap tall buildings in a single bound," says Samantha Heller, a nutritionist at NYU Medical Center.[59] Bars like Power Bar and Clif Bar were originally designed for endurance athletes, such as marathon runners or triathletes, who need something to replenish their energy after they hit the 15-mile mark, so they can make it to the finish line. Today, these high-carb, low-fat bars are marketed to lunchtime joggers and soccer moms, to help them fuel their personal workouts or get them through the day without stopping for a meal of real food.

> *Labeling a product an "energy food" is just a sly way of admitting it contains unnecessary calories.*

MYTH: Energy bars are better at improving workout performance than other pre-workout snacks.

WHY WE THINK THAT: We are always looking for ways to make our workouts easier and quicker while still wanting the most out of them. So, if a food item promises that, why not use it?

THE FACTS: Not according to research done at Ball State University in Muncie, Indiana. Scientists measured the performance of a group of trained cyclists during two-hour sessions fueled by energy bars, bagels, or fruit Newtons. No matter what the carb source, the athletes delivered identical performances. "There's absolutely no magic to these bars," says David Pearson, PhD, director of the university's Strength Research Laboratory.[60] "As long as the foods you eat are comparable in terms of carbs and calories, you're better off saving your money and paying 50 cents for a bagel instead of $2 for an energy bar."

In fact, eating an energy bar to help us get through our workout might be the reason we're gaining weight. "Most bars are the caloric equivalent of a two-and-a-half-mile run, and many people don't even burn off that many calories when they exercise," says Pearson.

> *Eating an energy bar to help us get through our workout might be the reason we're gaining weight.*

MYTH: Energy bars are a quick and easy way to get vitamins and minerals.

WHY WE THINK THAT: Since energy bars are represented to us as a high-quality food, we believe they must be filled with vitamins and minerals. Furthermore, since vitamins and minerals are good for us, we believe more is better.

THE FACTS: If we have at least one energy bar every day, there's a chance we're actually overloading on vitamins. "Some of these bars provide you with 100% of your RDA of vitamins and minerals, so if you eat one, take a vitamin pill, and also consume fortified breads and milk, you run the risk of ingesting mega-doses that could cause side effects," according to Tod Cooperman, MD, president of Consumerlab.com, an independent company that tests health, nutrition, and wellness products.[61] Too much vitamin A may weaken bones, excessive doses of vitamin C can cause diarrhea and canker sores, and overdoing vitamin B can result in nerve damage.

MYTH: Low-carb energy bars are low in carbs.

WHY WE THINK THAT: We believe low-carb energy bars are a healthy equivalent of a candy bar without having the load of sugar that comes with a candy bar.

THE FACTS: Many energy bars that promote the "low-carb life-style" in reality have plenty of carbs. In 2001, Consumerlab.com[62] tested thirty nutrition bars and found

> *Many energy bars that promote the "low-carb lifestyle" in reality have plenty of carbs.*

that half of them contained more carbs than they claimed. For example, one bar claimed it had only two grams of carbs, but had 22 grams instead. "Most of the carbohydrates in these products come from sweetening ingredients like glycerin, which manufacturers claim don't count as carbs because they don't impact blood sugar levels," says Dr. Cooperman. "But the reality is, they are still carbs, and they add up to 70% of a bar's total calories."

Energy-bar manufacturers are required by the FDA to list total carb counts on their nutrition labels. However, most low-carb bar manufacturers have found a loophole; they list only net carbs, which are actually grams of carbs minus grams of fiber and sugar alcohols. Meanwhile, their labeling information reveals the actual carb count to be five to nine times that amount. For example, an Atkins Advantage Chocolate Decadence bar says it has two grams of net carbs but actually it contains a total of 25 grams of carbs.

Net carbs are still carbohydrates but their appeal is that they make a food item appear lower in carbohydrates than it really is. Since the term *net carb* is not regulated by the FDA, it can mean whatever the manufacturer desires. Net carbs may have less impact on blood sugar levels but they still have an impact that can't be ignored. People who think net carbs don't count as calories in a weight-loss program are wrong. All carbohydrates are part of the entire food item and have calories that count.

"None of these so-called low-carb products are truly low-carb, and they may be loaded with fat, which is even worse," says Dr. Cooperman. Many bars have about

> *All carbohydrates are part of the entire food item and have calories that count.*

ten grams of fat, or about 15% of your RDA, which is the same as a Milky Way candy bar. "They can be high-fat candy bars in weight-loss packaging," says Lona Sandon, assistant professor of nutrition at the University of Texas Southwestern Medical Center in Dallas and a spokeswoman for the American Dietetic Association.

MYTH: Energy bars are a good fix for a no-time-for-lunch crunch.

WHY WE THINK THAT: We all have busy schedules, so, this way, we can skip mealtime without skipping a meal.

THE FACTS: A lot of us think grabbing an energy bar is better than skipping a meal, but experts say we should make this the exception, not the rule. These bars are appropriate in emergency situations but in reality are engineered foods. They usually don't contain enough calories to keep you full, so you may end up overeating later.[63] You're also missing out on healthier foods, such as fresh fruits and vegetables.

Energy bars should not routinely replace meals containing whole foods, especially fruits, vegetables, and whole grains, which

> *A diet rich in energy bars is often poor in variety.*

all contain fiber, vitamins, and phytochemicals. A diet rich in energy bars is often poor in variety. Energy bars come in a wide range of sizes, calorie levels, and specific carbohydrate, fat, and protein content. The scientific literature clearly documents that active individuals need carbohydrates to fuel the brain and muscles during exercise, and then need to replace their muscle glycogen after exercise. Therefore, during exercise, athletes need to consume energy bars or other foods that are high in carbohydrates. Bars and other foods with higher amounts of protein and fat will not provide an athlete with the fuel necessary to prevent fatigue and maintain blood glucose levels. In addition, bars and other foods with higher amounts of protein and fat will slow digestion; thus, an athlete may experience gastrointestinal distress while exercising.

In addition to higher carbohydrate needs, athletes also have slightly higher protein requirements than their sedentary counterparts. The higher protein needs of athletes have prompted manufacturers to boost the protein content of their products. However, protein is not normally used as a fuel source for activity, so a high-protein bar would not be a good choice prior to exercise or during exercise. However, after exercise, protein in combination with carbohydrate has been found to be beneficial in helping to enhance muscle glycogen replacement. Therefore, it would be appropriate to consume a bar or other food that contains carbohydrate and protein after exercise, to satisfy this need for both.

Athletes also require adequate amounts of fat, but fat consumed during exercise is not readily available for energy. Also, fat takes longer to digest so an athlete may experience intestinal discomfort after consuming a high-fat bar. Prior to exercise and during exercise, athletes should choose bars or other foods that contain no more than three to four grams of fat.

Notice that this answer addresses the needs of athletes, not sedentary individuals. Energy bars are meant to provide quick available

Energy bars are often high in calories.

energy during or shortly after a hard workout, so depleted carbohydrate resources can be replaced. Energy bars are often high in calories, and athletes need to remember that energy bars can significantly increase total daily caloric intake. Most bars contain 200-300 calories, so we need to be especially careful when using them regularly as snacks. Energy bars can be expensive and are not magic. The only "magic" about energy bars is that they are pre-wrapped, portable, and convenient. When used in sports situations, energy bars can be handy and provide necessary fuel for exercise. But for day-to-day snacking and meals, choose real foods for more nutrients and variety.

If you want to lose weight and think you'd like to try a meal-replacement product, first weigh the pros and cons. On the plus side, meal replacements:

- Are convenient
- Can save you time
- Are calorie- and portion-controlled
- Are often fortified with vitamins and minerals
- Often have a sweet taste that can satisfy a sweet tooth

On the downside, meal replacements:

- Can be expensive
- Often become boring because they don't come in many varieties. For example, Slim Fast® shakes come in only a few flavors.
- Might not satisfy your appetite in the way a meal would. Drinking a shake may not be as satisfying as eating a turkey sandwich.
- Sometimes leave a "vitamin" aftertaste. If you don't like the taste, you won't stick with the program and lose weight.

MYTH: Energy bars are a healthy "grab and go" snack.

WHY WE THINK THAT: The bars are advertised as providing energy, vitamins, and nutrition. All of that sounds healthy.

THE FACTS: These bars claim to be great "anytime" snacks, full of vitamins and minerals. And many of them deliver! Luna bars, for instance, contain 100% of the daily requirements of eleven different nutrients, from vitamin C to riboflavin and niacin. Zone Perfect bars have at least 200% of the daily requirement for vitamins C, E, and B_6. But nutrients aren't all these bars contain. "They're also chock-full of calories, sugar, and fat," says NYU nutritionist Heller. "The typical bar has about 230 calories, which is something between a snack and a small meal." You may find that you're even hungrier after eating an energy bar because refined carbohydrates cause blood sugar levels to rise in your body. When those sugar levels drop an hour later, you'll be ravenous.

Many of these products also contain seven to ten grams of fat, usually in the form of unhealthy, saturated fat or trans fatty acids. These fats are associated with an

These bars claim to be great "anytime" snacks, full of vitamins and minerals.

increased risk of cancer and heart disease. Companies must list the total amount of fat on the label. Be sure to check the label for the words "partially hydrogenated," which indicates the presence of trans fats.

Nutritionists agree that energy bars are no substitute for healthy, whole food, but there are times when fresh fruits, vegetables, and lean protein just aren't readily available. In those situations, an energy bar could be better than relying on what's in the nearest vending machine. If you're in a pinch, choose a bar that has less than six grams of fat, and fewer than three of those grams should be saturated. If you're just snacking, look for a bar with 150 calories or less, like Power Bar's Pria bar. Or, if you have a bar with more calories, eat just half of it.

Eating half of the bar is also smart when you need a pre-workout boost. Choose a classic, high-carb bar and you'll still get plenty of energizing carbs without the extra calories. If you're eating an energy bar instead of lunch, choose one with about 15 grams of protein and five grams of fiber. "Look for a product that has at least 200 to 400 calories, if the bar's at the lower end of that spectrum, have some fruit or celery or

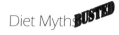

carrots sticks so you're not starving a couple of hours later," suggests nutritionist Liz Applegate, PhD, senior lecturer at the University of California-Davis.[64]

MYTH: Granola bars are a healthy alternative to a candy bar.
WHY WE THINK THAT: We often find granola cereals and granola snacks in health food stores or the health food section of the local grocery store.

THE FACTS: Granola bars contain around 200 calories and 15 grams or more of sugar, which is usually HFCS so the bars can stay good on the shelf for a long period of time. Calorie per calorie and sugar-gram per sugar-gram, granola isn't any better or different than a candy bar.

Calorie per calorie and sugar-gram per sugar-gram, granola isn't any better or different than a candy bar.

Energy Drinks

Now let us move on to enhanced fruit juices as an alternative replacement for plain juice or water. Advertisers push the idea that all we need to do is "drink to our health" and all will be well. Fruit juices with exotic supplements have spread from juice bars onto the supermarket shelves. But are these juices with feel-good extras really better for you than straight juice?

Fruit contains a vast array of nutrients — and most of us are not consuming enough fruits or vegetables. However, no single fruit or food will ever be the solution for all of our ailments, and — if anything — a diverse diet is best. These super-juices are pricey and come with a number of extraordinary and anecdotal health claims.

The newest juice to hit the market is kombucha, an ancient Chinese drink made from fermented tea. At the moment, young celebrities are raving about its medicinal properties. Advertising at its best. Among its purported health benefits, not yet evaluated or verified by the Food and Drug Administration, are that it speeds up metabolism, cleanses toxins from the bloodstream, reduces cholesterol levels, helps fight wrinkles, and boosts the immune system. Although frequently referred to as a mushroom, which it resembles, kombucha is not a mushroom; it's a colony of bacteria and yeast. Kombucha tea is made by adding the colony of bacteria and yeast to sugar and black or green tea and allowing the mix to ferment. There's no evidence that kombucha tea delivers on its health claims. At the same time, several cases of harm have been reported. Therefore, until definitive studies quantify the risks and benefits of kombucha tea, it's prudent to avoid it.[65]

It's both sad and astonishing to see sedentary people with a diet consisting of fast food and chips believing that a bottle of super-juice, endorsed by celebrities, will make them well.

> *There's no evidence that kombucha tea delivers on its health claims.*

Here are more myths surrounding energy drinks:

MYTH: Açai has more antioxidants than other fruits or juices.

WHY WE THINK THAT: If we watch daytime TV, we will see popular TV "Doctors" and other talk show hosts giving their approval of such exotic juices. We all know they don't lie.

THE FACTS: Açai is marketed under the names of Nu Açai and Guarana and contains 14% açai juice. It has 31% of the antioxidants of one red apple, yet it cost around $12 for 500 ml.

Amazonian açai, the cherry-sized purple berry fruit of the açai palm, deteriorates rapidly after harvest. This "amazing energy berry" is usually only available

> *Research confirms açai's high antioxidant levels, and lab studies suggest it may have anti-cancer and anti-inflammatory effects.*

outside the Amazon as juice or pulp that's been frozen, dried, or freeze-dried. Pulp can be added to juices or smoothies. Açai is reported to contain high levels of anthocyanins, compounds with antioxidant activity that are also responsible for its deep purple color. According to RioLife's marketing literature, açai was rated by a doctor on the TV show *Oprah* as "the #1 food for anti-aging benefits." Nu Fruits' website says açai berries have "six times the antioxidant level of blueberries" and touts them as a great source of essential fatty acids and energy, yet holds back from making specific health claims.

Research confirms açai's high antioxidant levels, and lab studies suggest it may have anti-cancer and anti-inflammatory effects, as well as a possible use in treating heart disease. However, these are the same claims other more common fruits have shown. These more common fruits are more available and cost less. Human studies on the health effects of açai are yet to be published.

MYTH: Goji berry juice is a cure all for chronic diseases.
WHY WE THINK THAT: Goji is among the many exotic fruits that claim to cure our chronic illnesses and we all want to just drink or eat away our aliments.

THE FACTS: Goji is marketed as Absolute Red NingXia Wolfberry and as Himalayan Goji Juice. Compared to an ordinary red apple, it has 34% of the antioxidants but it cost anywhere from $45 to $85 for just one liter.

The goji berry, or wolfberry, has been cultivated and eaten in Himalayan regions for centuries. Cellular and animal studies have investigated *If you take warfarin, see your doctor before drinking goji.* the impact of goji on the growth of human leukemia cells, aging, vision, insulin resistance, and infertility, among other things. Results from many show a positive effect, and it's suggested that polysaccharides unique to goji may play a key role. But good-quality clinical studies providing evidence for reported benefits in humans are lacking. If you take warfarin, see your doctor before drinking goji, as they may interact.

On a personal note: one of our family members has Type II diabetes and they are drinking this particular juice as a means of "curing" their affliction. You can't cure diabetes by drinking sugar water! It is like trying to put out a fire with gasoline.

MYTH: Mangosteen is good for everything from curing disease to losing weight.
WHY WE THINK THAT: If we can drink it or eat it instead of doing the hard, necessary work to be healthy and fit, we will do it.

THE FACTS: Mangosteen is a tropical fruit with a thick purplish rind and segmented white flesh. It's purported to contain more xanthones, a compound that may have antioxidant properties, than any other fruit. Mangosteen has only 17% of the nutritional value of an ordinary apple but costs up to $50 for 750 ml.

Literature claims that one bottle of mangosteen marketed as Xanberry has over double the antioxidant levels of goji juice.

Scientific research confirms that a variety of xanthones can be isolated from mangosteen plants and fruits. There are also a number of lab studies that suggest mangosteen extracts may have a use in the treatment of some cancers. However, clinical trials on real people are lacking and the claims come from the company, not outside, independent research labs.

MYTH: Noni juice is another miracle juice that cures everything from acne to cancer.

WHY WE THINK THAT: Another drink, another promise of an easy cure.

THE FACTS: Noni is a lime-green Polynesian tropical fruit that has a long history of medicinal use. Because the fruit in its natural state is bitter, it is often cut with copious amounts of more common fruit juices. This, of course, dilutes the properties of the straight noni juice. Typically it's the roots, bark, and leaves that are used for different remedies, usually by applying them externally to the skin or to wounds. Tahitian noni is considered the best of all the noni products sold. Of all the "miracle" juices sold, noni fares least well against the nutrition of an ordinary red apple. Noni has only 9% of the nutrition of a red delicious apple but cost anywhere from $40 to $60 for just one liter.

On a personal note: I work as a librarian and one of my coworkers was a noni distributor. She claimed it cured all of her aches and pains. She would take every opportunity to talk it up with coworkers and patrons. She even gave me a book written by a doctor that "proved" how wonderful it was. I pointed out to her that the book was written by a doctor employed by the company, commissioned by the company to do the studies, and the book was published by the noni company. What else was he going to say? They paid his salary![66]

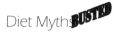

What to take away

- Energy bars and granola bars are glorified candy bars.
- Energy bars are often filled with nutritionally poor-quality ingredients.
- Energy bars are not a good replacement for a wholesome meal.
- Energy juices have the same problem as energy bars, just in a liquid.
- Exotic juices have no more antioxidant properties than ordinary, everyday, inexpensive fruits.

21. NUTRITION AND SEX

I'm at the age where food has taken the place of sex. In fact, I just had a mirror put over my kitchen table.
— Rodney Dangerfield

Nutrition has an effect on sex? Of course! Nutrition affects any aspect of physical performance. Our sexual health and enjoyment are directly related to our level of fitness and our nutritional intake. Almost all of us experience changes in our sexual health at one point or another in our lives, for any of many reasons, such as illness, disability, fatigue, obesity, low self-esteem, medications, recreational drugs, past sexual experiences, and loss of sexual interest in a partner. Proper management of life's uncertainties is essential for sexual health. In order to maintain sexual health, we need to feel desire and be desired. We need to have our body and mind in sync.

A healthy sex life requires good blood circulation, which is a result of good nutrition. Sexual vitality decreases with malnutrition. Poor

Nutrition has an effect on sex? Of course!

nutrition decreases blood circulation by allowing plaque to build up in the arteries. Good blood circulation allows adequate nutrition and oxygen to go to all of the body's organs. Proper blood circulation increases sensitivity in the penis and in the clitoris, improves physical vitality and stamina, and helps maintain good hormonal function.

A healthy cardiovascular system should be one major focus of any diet. Maintaining good circulation and a healthy weight will lead to improved sexual function and health. Protein intake from sources such as eggs, fish, meat, or poultry has been proven to increase libido (sex drive). Cholesterol level and ratio are also important. If HDL levels are low, sexual performance and vitality can be affected. On the other hand, if LDL levels are too high, decreased sensitivity in the genitals will result, therefore decreasing pleasure. A balanced diet is extremely important to optimize sexual responsiveness and performance by maintaining good blood circulation, hormonal balance, and a manageable weight.

Protein, carbohydrates, fats, and water all have a role in sexual function. Our brain operates on signals that are transmitted by brain chemicals, many of which are formed from amino acids found in protein. When we ingest good sources of protein, these neurotransmitters are formed, brain function is stimulated, and we feel more alert and ready for sexual action.

Carbohydrates tend to be a sedative. A meal that is lacking in protein and high in carbohydrates can make us drowsy. The consequence is an initial sharp rise in blood glucose followed by a rapid decline, causing lethargy. While we should eat both carbs and protein at an evening meal, try adding a bit more protein in place of that extra helping of carbohydrate. It helps balance our meal and our frame of mind.

> *Protein, carbohydrates, fats, and water all have a role in sexual function.*

Fats can slow us down. A high-fat diet can very quickly lead to excess weight, and this can cause the buildup of plaque inside critical blood vessels, which obstructs normal blood flow. Adequate blood flow to the genitals is an important aspect of sexual response. For good sexual performance and overall health, we need to limit our consumption of trans fats and keep healthier fats in balance with the rest of our diet.

Water is our most critical nutrient. If we're not replenishing our fluid stores, we're not going to feel ready for anything. An unbalanced diet, lacking enough water and containing inferior sources of nutrients will make a person grouchy, tired, and not at all in the mood or ready to feel romantic.

An excess of any macronutrient will cause weight gain and that will cause insulin resistance, arterial inflammation, and pressure on the joints. All of this impedes movement, blood circulation, and breathing. Without a good supply of oxygen in the blood to our brain and other vital organs, including the genitals, our energy levels drop and our desire for physical and emotional intimacy decreases.

MYTH: Aphrodisiacs work and increase desire.

WHY WE THINK THAT: We all like the notion that the mysteries of sex and love can be controlled with exotic foods and mystical potions.

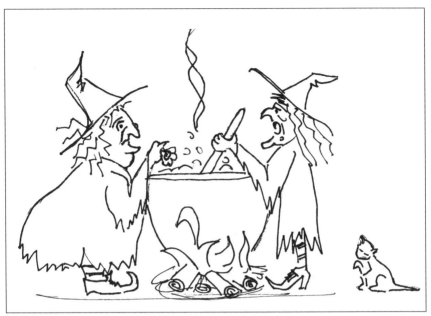

Eye of newt, wart of toad, tongue of snake. What we women will do to stay sexy and desirable!

THE FACTS: People like the concept of an aphrodisiac. The FDA defines an aphrodisiac as a food, drink, drug, scent, or device that claims to increase sexual desire and improve or enhance performance. Seafood is one of the best-known aphrodisiacs. Fish are believed to stimulate the brain and sexual function. Shellfish, such as oysters and clams, are among the favorites because of their high levels of zinc. Foods with high zinc content stimulate male prostate function as well as male fertility, testosterone production, and sex drive. Seaweeds, which are rich in minerals, also enhance libido.

Low levels of zinc can cause impotence, low sperm count, and loss of sexual interest. However, zinc should not be taken excessively

Seafood is one of the best-known aphrodisiacs.

because it can suppress the immune system and reduce absorption of necessary minerals, such as copper and manganese. Vitamin C deficiency can lead to male infertility. Vitamin E, also known as the "sex vitamin," supposedly increases the hardness and duration of an erection.

The amino acid arginine boosts sperm production. This amino acid is found in many foods, such as milk, meat, chicken, and fish. Amino acids are the building blocks of proteins, enzymes, and hormones, and are known to play a key role in physiological functions. Arginine is important in the process of neurotransmission, immune function, the relaxation of blood vessels, and the flow of blood to the male and female sex organs. In the body, arginine is required for the synthesis of nitric oxide, a natural compound that enables the arterial system to retain its elasticity and thus its ability to increase the flow of blood to the tissues of the body. Arginine, via nitric oxide, allows the capillaries to expand and contract, thus moving blood through the blood vessels.

Chocolate contains phenylethylamine and serotonin, which are mood-lifting agents found naturally in the human brain. They are released into the nervous system by the brain when we are happy and when we are experiencing feelings of love, passion, or lust. Phenylethylamine and serotonin cause rapid mood changes, a rise in blood pressure, an increase in heart rate, and induce feelings of well-being bordering on the type of euphoria often associated with being in love.

Chocolate contains mood-lifting agents found naturally in the human brain.

Eating chocolate also releases phenylethylamine and serotonin into the blood system, producing those same euphoric effects, plus chocolate can provide a substantial energy boost, thus increasing stamina. These effects probably caused chocolate to gain its reputation as an aphrodisiac. Now we know why chocolate is a favorite gift for Valentine's Day!

Recent research suggests that women are more susceptible to the effects of phenylethylamine and serotonin than men. The famous lover Casanova is said to have consumed chocolate before frolicking with his conquests, but there's no mention of him actually sharing it. The greatest and most reliable aphrodisiac, however, is between our ears. A healthy, well-nourished mind provides the means to provide and fill the imagination for a healthy sex life.

MYTH: Aphrodisiacs must be eaten.

WHY WE THINK THAT: Many of the aphrodisiacs we know of are foods we eat.

THE FACTS: True. Many foods do seem to have an effect on our sexual responses. "Different foods have different nutrients and substances that affect the body physiologically in different ways, that's why different foods work for different stages," says clinical sexologist Ava Cadell, PhD. "Some foods lower inhibitions, some get the blood flowing directly to the genitalia, and some foods release happy hormones."[67]

There are foods that are good for flirting, there are foods that are good for seduction, and there are foods that are good for performance.

Flirt-friendly foods include:

- Chili peppers. Spicy foods get the heart pumping, raise the heart rate, and induce sweating.
- Bananas. They contain chemicals that have a mood-lifting effect on the brain, which raises self-confidence.
- Carrots. Their phallic appearance and high-fiber content induce sexual desire.

Aphrodisiacs can help trigger the release of sex hormones, provide a quick energy boost, and increase blood flow to the genitals to get the body "in the mood." Visually erotic foods automatically set our brain in motion. Oysters, fresh figs, and carrots are foods that resemble the genitalia, just to name a few.

Aphrodisiacs can help trigger the release of sex hormones, provide a quick energy boost, and increase blood flow to the genitals.

Certain foods stimulate the release of hormones such as testosterone, which makes women more sexually adventurous and aggressive.

Foods for seduction include:

- Seafood. Shrimp and other types of seafood are high in iodine and vital to the thyroid gland, which is necessary for energy.
- Chocolate. It provides a jolt of caffeine along with other sexually stimulating chemicals.

- Ginger. This root increases blood flow to the genitals in both men and women.
- Olives. Green ones are believed to make men more virile, while black ones increase women's sex drive.
- Tomatoes. Termed "love apples" by the Puritans, tomatoes have a reputation as a sexual stimulant.
- Apples. Since Adam and Eve, this fruit has been linked to sexual desire.
- Asparagus. Long and phallic-looking, it's rich in potassium, phosphorus, calcium, and vitamin E, all of which aid in hormone production and raising energy levels.

Foods for sexual performance:

- Blueberries. Often called "nature's little blue pills" because of their similarities to Viagra. They're loaded with soluble fiber, which push excess cholesterol through the digestive system before it can be broken down, absorbed, and deposited in the arteries. Blueberries have compounds that relax blood vessels, thus improving circulation throughout the body. The benefit of lower cholesterol and improved blood flow is more blood flow to the genitals during sex.

> *Blueberries are often called "nature's little blue pills."*

- Whole-grain, unrefined breads and cereals. These are rich in niacin, a vitamin that's essential for the secretion of histamine. Our bodies need histamine in order to control and trigger explosive orgasms!

In the final stage of the sexual experience, just the scent of some aphrodisiacs can be enough to increase sexual arousal and enhance performance.

"Depending on where you are in your relationship, you may want to use different food odors and tastes, since 90% of taste is smell, to get the different responses you're looking for," says Alan R. Hirsch, MD, neurological director of the Smell and Taste Treatment and Research Foundation in Chicago.[68]

In a study that looked at which scents stimulated sexual arousal, Dr. Hirsch found that every food aroma tested triggered a sexual response in men, and some foods had more dramatic effects than others. Cheese

Every food aroma tested triggered a sexual response in men.

pizza increased penile blood flow by 5%, buttered popcorn by 9%, and lavender scent and pumpkin pie by 40%. This should be a good incentive for men to learn to make natural cheese pizza, healthy popcorn, and homemade pumpkin pie all illuminated with a lavender scented candle!

In comparison, floral perfume only prompted a 3% increase in blood flow to the penis among men. Among women, the smell of men's cologne actually lowered blood flow to the vagina. So much for expensive bottles of colognes and perfumes. A cheese-pizza or pumpkin-pie perfume might be more effective and less expensive!

The study found that the combined scent of lavender and pumpkin pie was also a powerful sexual stimulant for women, but the combination of the scents of the

The combined scent of lavender and pumpkin pie was a powerful sexual stimulant for women.

licorice-flavored candy, Good & Plenty, and cucumber caused the greatest increase in blood flow to the vaginal area. The study also found that some food odors actually inhibited sexual desire in women, such as the smell of cherries and the odor of barbeque or roasting meat, but these foods did not decrease men's desire.

The bottom line: whether a man or woman, put a dab of lavender or pumpkin pie behind your ears if you want to attract a potential mate.

MYTH: Semen is low-carb.

WHY WE THINK THAT: We think that most of our body fluids are made of protein and various nutrients.

THE FACTS: True! Semen is 150 mg of protein, 11 mg of carbohydrates, 6 mg fat, 3 mg cholesterol, 7% US RDA potassium and 3% US RDA copper and zinc. Therefore, semen is mostly a protein and therefore, low-carb.

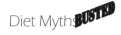

MYTH: Eating broccoli or asparagus is healthy and will not affect the taste of semen.

WHY WE THINK THAT: We are so focused on how healthy our diet is when it goes into our body, but not so much on how it affects the fluids that leave our body.

THE FACTS: Semen has a naturally slightly bitter taste. Eating some foods, such as broccoli and asparagus, and drinking coffee can exacerbate that taste. While we don't need to eliminate these healthy foods from our diet, we might want to be careful about when we consume them. On the other hand, drinking or eating sweet fruits, such as pineapple, oranges, and bananas, will sweeten the taste.

MYTH: Women have their own unique taste, so foods don't affect them.

WHY WE THINK THAT: Women, unlike men, don't eject a substantial amount of fluid during sex, so we think as long as we are clean, we will taste fine.

THE FACTS: Sushi and soy sauce will leave a woman tasting salty. Some foods, such as broccoli, asparagus, and cauliflower, will leave a more bitter taste as well as a

> *Any fruit, especially melons, will make either gender's secretions taste sweeter and lighter.*

more pungent smell. Heavy spices, such as onion and garlic, will also leave a stronger taste and smell. Pineapple, kiwi, melon, and strawberries will leave women tasting and smelling sweet. One AA devotee shared this little tip; "I haven't had anything to drink but pineapple juice and water for years, and every man I am with has said I taste like nectar."[69] Any fruit, especially melons, will make either gender's secretions taste sweeter and lighter. For both sexes, the effects take only a few hours to manifest themselves. Eat broccoli, asparagus, and cauliflower because they are healthy and tasty, but do plan accordingly for your sexual activitics!

MYTH: Green M&Ms make you desire sex.

WHY WE THINK THAT: We all remember hearing that old tale when we were in grade school.

THE FACTS: If we believe they will make us horny, they will, and if we believe they won't, they won't. Ah, the power of the mind and the placebo effect can work wonders. However, since M&Ms contain chocolate, any color just might work!

> *The power of the mind and the placebo effect can work wonders.*

MYTH: Drinking alcohol will improve a person's sexual performance.

WHY WE THINK THAT: Alcohol in our system often makes us feel we can do anything and be anybody.

THE FACTS: In small amounts, alcohol might reduce inhibitions, but too much alcohol acts as a depressant and can deaden sexual sensations. Alcohol also dulls higher brain functions that control sexual behavior and judgment. Although it may put us in the mood, alcohol paradoxically inhibits our ability to perform and enjoy sex.

MYTH: What we eat really doesn't affect our sex life.

WHY WE THINK THAT: Since we know that the greatest influence on sex is the brain, we think we can eat what we want.

THE FACTS: True, the brain is the center of interest and desire. However, if we don't fuel it properly, it won't work properly, nor will the rest of our body. Humankind has three basic instincts: we must survive, we must eat, and we must procreate. Since one instinct feeds the other and they all contribute to our survival, it is hard to separate nutrition and sex. A poor diet that consists of non-nutritious foods can lead to erectile dysfunction (ED) in men and decreased libido in women. Refined flours, sugars, and trans fats cause an increase in LDL-cholesterol and narrowing of the arteries. Researchers at the University of South Carolina School of Medicine in Columbia examined the LDL-cholesterol levels and sex lives of 3,250 men over age 24.[70] They found that as a man's LDL-cholesterol went up, so did his likelihood of suffering from ED. LDL-cholesterol narrows the arteries that nourish the heart and increases the risk of heart attack. LDL also narrows the arteries that carry blood into the penis, which contributes to erectile dysfunction. These arteries are some of the smallest, and are the first to jam up with plaque.

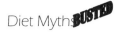

In women, the arteries that go to the clitoris are the ones that will close up with plaque, leading to desensitization. This is particularly unfortunate for women, because unlike men, the sole purpose of this organ is for pleasure. The clitoris contains between 7,000 to 10,000 nerve endings that need to be supplied with blood in order to function.

As a man's LDL-cholesterol went up, so did his likelihood of suffering from ED

Just something to think about: if we continue to feed our children nutritiously inadequate food, not only are they destined not to live as long as the previous generation, but they may also lack the desire to produce future generations.

MYTH: Soy is a healthy food and will improve a man's sexual function.

WHY WE THINK THAT: Healthy foods are good for all aspects of our lives.

THE FACTS: Soy foods are a great source of protein and, eaten in moderation as part of a balanced diet, will not adversely affect a man's sexual function. However, since soy products contain isoflavones, eating lots of soy products every day can potentially lower a man's testosterone levels and, thus, his sexual desires. So have a soy protein shake after a hard workout a couple of times a week. Just don't have them every day. In this situation, men should opt for whey protein as a first choice.

MYTH: Good nutrition leads to better sex.

WHY WE THINK THAT: Just as a car will run better with good fuel and maintenance, we will too.

THE FACTS: A myth that is not a myth! Foods that are high in vitamin A, such as fish, eggs,

Good nutrition leads to better sex. True!

cheese, yogurt, green leafy vegetables, and yellow fruits, help maintain our sex hormones. Foods that are high in vitamin B_1, such as whole, unrefined grains, rice, pineapple, beans, asparagus, and nuts, are essential for energy production and it takes energy to engage in sexual activity! Vitamin B_3, also called niacin, helps increase blood flow to our organs,

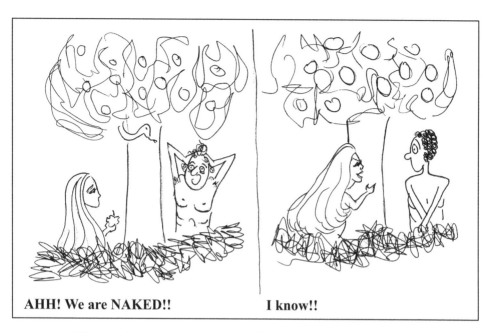

AHH! We are NAKED!!

I know!!

extremities, and our brain. We need all of those parts of our bodies to have an adequate blood supply in order to perform sexually and enjoy it. Foods high in vitamin B_3 are broccoli, yogurt, lean meats, fish, and chicken. Adequate amounts of vitamin C are essential for healthy sexual activity. Vitamin C helps with energy production in the formation of blood cells, in the absorption of iron, and in oxygenation of the tissues. Blood cells carry oxygen, hormones, and nutrients to the organs, glands, and tissues of the body. Healthy hormone production influences our sexual abilities. Our immune system is strengthened by vitamin C, and that protects against stress and disease as well as keeping our joints limber and active. Good sources of vitamin C are tomatoes, strawberries, and citrus fruits.

What to take away

- A healthy diet leads to a healthy libido (sex drive).
- Foods that narrow the arteries to our heart narrow the arteries to our genitals.
- The best and most powerful aphrodisiac is the brain.

22. Pregnancy and Nutrition

Q: Our baby was born last week. When will my wife begin to feel and act normal again?
A: When the kids are in college.

— Unknown

MYTH: Eating for two is necessary when pregnant.

WHY WE THINK THAT: Since we are carrying another human inside of us, we need to feed them as well as ourselves.

THE FACTS: Energy requirements vary among individuals. Unfortunately, the idea that pregnancy is an ice-cream free-for-all is a nutrition myth. We need to eat with the understanding that we are providing the building material for the development of another human being, along with our own nutritional requirements. We are not eating for ourselves and another full-sized human. It is generally recommended that pregnant women increase their daily intake by 100 calories in the first trimester and 300 calories in the second and third trimesters. An extra snack before bedtime, such as a serving of fruit, a serving of milk or yogurt, and a few whole grain crackers, is often enough. A daily prenatal multivitamin supplement is often recommended during pregnancy, but not a daily bowl of ice cream!

The idea that pregnancy is an ice-cream free-for-all is a nutrition myth.

Researchers have found that when women gain more than 53 lbs. while pregnant they produce heavier babies who have a higher predisposition to becoming obese children and adults.[71]

MYTH: Salt will make you swell up.

WHY WE THINK THAT: Salt makes us thirsty, and so we drink more water. We also believe that since salt makes us retain water, we will swell up.

THE FACTS: Even when pregnant, salt is an essential nutrient but should not be eaten in excessive amounts. We can salt our food to taste and should read the labels on food packages carefully to watch for hidden sources of sodium.

MYTH: The baby will take what it needs from the mother's body.

WHY WE THINK THAT: Women have been getting pregnant for eons. Just let nature take its course.

THE FACTS: The baby is being built from protein, a nutrient our body uses to build tissues. Our body does not store extra quantities of protein to use to build a baby. If we do not eat adequate amounts of protein, our own health will suffer

> *If we do not eat adequate amounts of protein, our own health will suffer as our body begins to break down our muscle tissues to develop and feed the baby.*

as our body begins to break down our muscle tissues to develop and feed the baby. If we want to stay healthy and have a healthy baby, the only source of protein our baby has is from the food we eat.

MYTH: If we eat less, the baby will take nourishment from the extra fat we have.

WHY WE THINK THAT: Part of this is wishful thinking. We also know that fat is an energy source; so we think that if it feeds us, it should feed our baby.

THE FACTS: The baby is being built from protein, not fat. Fat is how our body stores calories, the main source of energy for our body. It cannot be made into protein to build the baby's tissues. If we don't eat enough protein, our body will have to break down our muscles to provide the necessary protein to nourish the baby, leaving us sick and weak.

MYTH: Eating a low-fat diet will keep the extra weight off during pregnancy.

WHY WE THINK THAT: We believe that if we avoid fat, we can avoid gaining extra weight, even when pregnant.

> *Eating too much of anything, including fat, is the problem.*

THE FACTS: Fat is an essential macronutrient. Fat is no more a culprit for being overweight than carbohydrates or proteins. Eating fat is not the problem; eating too much of anything, including fat, is the problem, even when pregnant. Too much food of any type will be stored by our body as fat. Low-fat diets can be dangerous because most foods that are considered fattening are good sources of protein, such as eggs, meats, and cheese. A diet low in protein is dangerous during pregnancy.

MYTH: Pregnant women should avoid caffeine.

WHY WE THINK THAT: We are afraid that since caffeine can temporarily raise our blood pressure, it will also raise the baby's blood pressure.

THE FACTS: Pregnant women can take caffeine in moderation (one to two cups per day). Many women find they experience changes in taste during pregnancy and don't want to drink tea or coffee. For those who continue to enjoy their tea and coffee, most physicians and researchers agree that moderate amounts of coffee will have no adverse effects on the outcome of the pregnancy or the infant's health.

MYTH: I can get iron from meat sources only.

WHY WE THINK THAT: We hear a lot about how much iron is in meats, but we tend to be unaware of the other sources.

THE FACTS: A balanced diet that includes foods high in iron can help ensure that we are consuming enough iron throughout our pregnancy. The United States' recommended daily allowance (RDA) for iron is 27 milligrams for pregnant women and 15 milligrams for breastfeeding women. Eating at least three servings of iron-rich foods a day will help ensure that we are getting thirty milligrams of iron in our daily diet. One of the best ways to get iron in our diet is to consume a highly fortified breakfast cereal such as Total, which contains eighteen milligrams of iron per serving. Note that iron intake is not equal to iron absorption. Absorption of iron into the body is greatest from meat.

Eat at least three servings of iron-rich foods a day.

The best sources of iron include enriched grain products, lean meat, poultry, fish, and leafy green vegetables. Good animal-protein sources of iron include lean beef, chicken, clams, crab, egg yolk, fish, lamb, liver, oysters, pork, sardines, shrimp, turkey, and veal. Good vegetable sources of iron include black-eyed peas, broccoli, Brussels sprouts, collard and turnip greens, lima beans, sweet potatoes, and spinach. Dry beans and peas, lentils, and soybeans are good legume sources of iron. Good fruit sources of iron include berries, apricots, dried fruits (such as prunes, raisins, and apricots), grapes, grapefruit, oranges, plums, prune juice, and watermelon. You can also get iron from enriched rice and pasta, soft pretzels, and whole-grain, enriched or fortified breads and cereals. Other foods that contain iron are molasses, peanuts, pine nuts, and seeds from pumpkin and squash.

MYTH: Food cravings will interfere with good nutrition.

WHY WE THINK THAT: Well, pickles and ice cream may not be the most appetizing meal, but it won't hurt.

THE FACTS: If you give in to cravings for junk food, then you will gain unnecessary weight and not provide adequate nutrition for you and your baby. When I was pregnant with my daughter, I craved apples and white cheeses. With my son, I craved green peppers and avocados. The only person who seemed to suffer from my cravings was my husband; he just didn't have the same passion for apples, cheese, green peppers, and avocados that I did!

Food cravings during pregnancy are normal. Although there is no widely accepted explanation for food cravings, almost two-thirds of all pregnant women have them. If you develop a sudden urge for a certain food, go ahead and indulge your craving if it provides energy or an essential nutrient. But if your craving persists and prevents you from getting other essential nutrients in your diet, try to create more of a balance in your daily diet during pregnancy.

Food cravings during pregnancy are normal.

During pregnancy, taste for certain foods may change. It is not unusual to develop a dislike for foods you were fond of before you became pregnant, and it is not unusual to crave foods you once didn't like much. Some women feel strong urges to eat non-food items, such as ice, laundry starch, dirt, clay, chalk, ashes, or paint chips. This is called *pica*, and it may be associated with iron-deficiency anemia or other

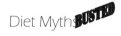

health problems. Such cravings can be harmful to both you and your baby, so don't give in to them. Tell your health care provider if you have these non-food cravings.

Ask your health care provider for advice if you have any problems that prevent you from eating balanced meals and gaining weight properly. No matter how strong your desire may be, avoid foods considered health risks for pregnant women and developing babies. These include:

> *Ask your health care provider for advice if you have any problems that prevent you from eating balanced meals and gaining weight properly.*

- Raw and undercooked seafood, meat, and eggs
- Unpasteurized milk and any foods made from it
- Unpasteurized juice
- Raw vegetable sprouts, including alfalfa, clover, and radish
- Herbal teas
- Alcohol

What to take away

- When pregnant, eat normally; don't eat for two full-sized adults.
- Just as a healthy diet affects the mother's health, a healthy diet also affects the health of the fetus.
- Eat a good balance of macronutrients.

23. FEEDING BABIES AND CHILDREN

I always wondered why babies spend so much time sucking their thumbs. Then I tasted baby food.

— Robert Orben

As a child my family's menu consisted of two choices: take it or leave it.

— Buddy Hackett

Without question, the best food for a baby is human breast milk. Just as cow's milk is made for cows and lion's milk is made for lions, human milk is ready-made for humans. And what goes into the mother comes out in her milk. A diet that is rich in wholesome foods will produce superior milk and a diet of junk food will produce inferior milk.

The number-one predictor of whether a child will have a weight problem is how physically fit or unfit the parents are. If one parent is unfit, a child has a 40% chance of being overweight. If both parents are unfit, that statistic jumps to 80-90%.[72] The eating habits that children learn early in life from their parents form the basis of how they will eat for the rest of their lives and it will have a lasting impact on their health.

> The number-one predictor of whether a child will have a weight problem is how physically fit or unfit the parents are.

Once a baby is ready for solid food, it's time to rethink everything we thought we knew about feeding babies. It turns out that most advice we get about starting infants on solid foods, even from pediatricians, is more myth than science. For instance, rice cereal may not be the best first food, and introducing peanut butter doesn't have to wait until after a baby's first birthday. Offering fruits before vegetables won't breed a sweet tooth, and spices are just fine. "There's a bunch of mythology out there about this," says Dr. David Bergman, a Stanford University professor of pediatrics.[73] "There's not much evidence to support any particular way of doing things."

Research increasingly suggests that a child's first experiences with food shape their later eating habits. Debunking the myths and broadening our babies' palates may help children battle obesity later on in life. The federal government has given little attention to how to introduce young children to solid food, and dietary guidelines apply only to children two years old and older.

It is both easy and hard to change how we think about feeding our babies. Easy, because four- to six-month-olds can eat many of the

A child's first experiences with food shape their later eating habits.

same things we do and they haven't yet learned to be finicky. Hard, because it's tough to convince nervous parents that feeding children regular food is okay. Most parents are told by their doctors to start rice cereal at six months, and then slowly progress to simple vegetables, mild fruits, and finally, pasta and meat. Rachel Brandeis, a spokeswoman for the American Dietetic Association, says, "Babies start with a very clean palate and it's your job to mold it."[74]

In America, ethnic foods and spicy foods containing, for example, curry, cinnamon, and tahini, are ignored by parents who are told to avoid foods such as nuts and seafood for at least the first year of their child's life. Parents elsewhere in the world take a more casual approach. They start their babies on heartier, more flavorful fare such as meats in African countries, fish and radishes in Japan, and artichokes and tomatoes in France. Children over six months of age can handle almost anything, with a few exceptions. If allergies run in your family, you may need to be a little more vigilant, introducing one food at a time while you watch for any problems. And always make sure the food isn't a choking hazard.

Nancy Butte, a pediatrics professor at Baylor College of Medicine, found that many strongly held assumptions, such as the need to offer foods in a particular order or to delay the introduction of allergenic foods, have little scientific basis. Take rice cereal, for example. Conventional American wisdom says it's the best first food. But Butte says iron-rich meat, which often is one of the last foods American parents introduce, would be a better choice.[75]

Dr. David Ludwig of Children's Hospital in Boston, a specialist in pediatric nutrition, says some studies suggest rice and other highly processed grain cereals actually could be among the worst foods for infants. "These foods are, in a certain sense, no different from adding sugar to formula. They digest very rapidly in the body, become a sugar, raising blood sugar and insulin levels, and could contribute to later health problems, including obesity," he says. The lack of variety in the American approach could also be a problem. Exposing infants to more foods may help them adapt to different foods later, which Ludwig says may be crucial to getting older children to eat healthier.[76]

Parents' fear of food allergies is much of the reason for the bland-food approach to feeding babies. For decades, doctors have said that the best way to prevent allergies is to give infants only bland foods, avoiding seasonings, citrus, nuts, and certain seafood. But Butte's review found no evidence that children without family histories of food allergies benefit from this. Butte suspects that avoiding certain foods or eating bland diets could actually make allergies more likely. Some exposure might be a good thing.

It turns out that spices are just fine for babies. Science is catching up with the folklore that babies in

Spices are just fine for babies.

the womb and those who are breast-fed develop a taste for whatever a mother eats. Experts say that if a mother enjoys lots of basil, her baby might too.

That's been Maru Mondragon's experience.[77] She allowed herself plenty of spicy foods while pregnant with her youngest son, 21-month-old Russell, but not while carrying his three-year-old brother Christian. Christian avoids spices while his younger brother snacks on jalapeños and demands hot salsa on everything. Parents should view this as an opportunity to encourage children to indulge in a variety of different foods and develop healthy eating habits while introducing them to their culture and heritage, and to other foods.

MYTH: Young children are more finicky than older children.

WHY WE THINK THAT: Go to any restaurant or family gathering, and we often see children in highchairs squirming around and turning their noses up at all sorts of foods.

THE FACTS: Surprisingly, it is easier to encourage younger children rather than older kids to try new foods. Younger children don't know to be finicky, so smile and be positive when introducing a new food, and then the child will more

> It is easier to encourage younger children rather than older kids to try new foods.

than likely believe they will enjoy the food. Don't give up if your child doesn't like a food when he or she tries it for the first time. Keep in mind that children learn new food preferences through repeated exposure, and it could take eight to ten tries. Use cookie-cutter shapes to make eating vegetables more fun. Or make funny faces or other designs on plates with a new vegetable; for example, make a smiley face out of corn or peas.

MYTH: Preschoolers should drink whole milk.

WHY WE THINK THAT: We believe growing children need many sources of fats.

THE FACTS: Whole milk gives children under two years increased energy and the fat they need for brain development. After age two, children can have low-fat milk as long as their diet is more varied and they get essential fats from other foods. If there are no other fats in the diet, have the child drink whole milk. Be sure your child is eating from all the major food groups and include nuts, nut butters, avocados, and fish in their diet.

MYTH: My preschooler will outgrow his/her food allergy.

WHY WE THINK THAT: We see our children outgrow many common food allergies so we think they will outgrow them all.

THE FACTS: By the age of three years, most young children do outgrow common food allergies, such as milk, soy, and eggs, but they may not outgrow other allergies, such as peanuts or tree nuts. If you are uneasy about new foods, don't introduce more than one on the same day. If your child has no reaction to a new food after eating it for a few days, then you can include it in your child's diet and offer another new food. In countries other than the United States, children eat the same foods as adults. Always discuss any allergy concerns with your child's pediatrician.

MYTH: Fruit drinks have vitamins and minerals, so preschoolers can drink all they want.
WHY WE THINK THAT: We want our children to eat, and they will eat if they like what we give them. As long as we think it is healthy, we believe it will be fine.

THE FACTS: Many fruit drinks do have added vitamins and minerals, but they also contain a lot of calories from sugar or other sweeteners, and they lack fiber. Associating quenching thirst with drinking sweet beverages can create a very unhealthy habit for children. It can desensitize them to sweets, so they will crave more sweets to satisfy their desires. This means that they will tend to fill up on foods that contain nutrient-deficient calories, which will increase their risk for obesity and other chronic ailments later on.

The best way to get vitamins and minerals into your child's diet is with whole fruits and vegetables. Not only do whole fruits and vegetables contain essential vitamins and *The best way to get vitamins and minerals into your child's diet is with whole fruits and vegetables.* minerals, they also contain fiber. The healthiest beverages for children are water, milk, and limited amounts of 100% fruit juice. To cut calories and sugar in juice and wean children off of them, water it down to a 50:50 ratio one-half water, one-half juice. Use seltzer to create a fizzy treat, or freeze juice in ice-cube trays and add these juice cubes to water.

MYTH: Children need red meat a few times a week to get enough iron.
WHY WE THINK THAT: We know that red meat is a good source of iron, and growing children need iron. We tend to be unfamiliar with other iron sources. *Children can get adequate iron from many other foods*

THE FACTS: Iron is a critical nutrient for growth and development, and red meat is an excellent source, so, by all means, feed children red meat now and then. However, red meat is not the only source of iron. Children can get adequate iron from many other foods, such as eggs, fish, poultry, beans, whole-grain or enriched cereal, bread, and dried fruit. Keeping their diet varied is also important. Don't let kids fill up on milk before eating red meat, fish, or poultry. Although an excellent source of many nutrients, milk does not contain iron, and the calcium and phosphorus in milk can impair iron absorption. It is interesting to note that the kosher and halal laws followed by devout Jews and Muslims prohibit the drinking of milk with meat.

MYTH: Children should be taught to clean their plates.

WHY WE THINK THAT: Who hasn't grown up with the mantras "clean your plate; I didn't work hard just to have you throw this away!" or "clean your plate; there are starving children in [name a country] who would give anything to have your dinner!" Believe me, when I was a child, if I could have given my butterbeans or my liver-and-onions to someone, anywhere, I would have! We want our children to appreciate what we give them, and we don't want them to feel deprived.

THE FACTS: Young children usually stop eating when they feel full and, as parents, we shouldn't override these natural eating cues.

Young children usually stop eating when they feel full.

When I nursed my children, I let them feed till they pushed me away. Sometimes they nursed for a few minutes, and other times I thought they would never let go. Consequently, when they moved on to solid food, they ate until they were full. Sometimes they ate very little and sometimes they ate quite a bit more. I remember when our daughter was young; I gave her a bowl of ice cream. She ate what she wanted and left half of it in the bowl. It was easy enough to put the bowl back in the freezer for another time. Today, both are adults and very physically active; our daughter is a personal trainer and our son is on a rowing team. Needless to say, when they come home to visit, meals are an event!

Adult-sized portions can overwhelm a child, so when feeding children, serve them small portions, and don't offer additional helpings unless they ask for more, then give out even smaller portions. Serve nutritious foods at the beginning of the meal, and be sure your child doesn't fill up with beverages. When eating out at a restaurant, it isn't healthy or necessary for children to have unlimited soda-pop refills, an easy way to overload them on sugar.

Encouraging children to eat more than they want can lead to negative eating behaviors in later years. Provide healthy nutritious meals and snacks, but allow your child to stop eating when satisfied. If a child asks for a snack, and you offer an apple or small box of raisins but they refuse it or ask for a candy bar instead, then they are not hungry. If they say they are thirsty, and you offer water or milk but they refuse the offer or ask for soda pop instead, they are not thirsty.

> *Encouraging children to eat more than they want can lead to negative eating behaviors in later years.*

MYTH: An overweight child needs to be on a diet.

WHY WE THINK THAT: If our child is overweight, we feel we need to take action. We are conditioned to believe diets work, so we believe they will work for our child.

THE FACTS: Overweight children should not be on diets such as those we see portrayed in magazines or popularized by celebrities. They should be fed like the preschooler or child that they are, not like teenagers or adults. If a child is overweight, provide him or her with healthy, well-balanced meals and snacks from whole, natural, real foods and limit nutritionally deficient, calorie-dense foods. Avoid all-you-can-eat buffets and unlimited soda-pop refills. Provide lots of opportunities for physical activity as an alternative form of entertainment instead of focusing on food. Use trips to the zoo, hands-on museums, or the park as incentives for good grades or behavior, not food.

Guidelines from the American Academy of Pediatrics state that the goal for all children ages two to seven years should be weight maintenance, not weight loss. This is accomplished by portioning out foods before serving them to children. This puts the parent in control of what and how much the child eats. Everyone in the family should eat the same healthy meals and snacks. Overweight children should never be made to feel they are being denied foods that others in the family are allowed to

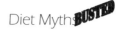

eat. In order to change an overweight child's behavior, the entire family must adopt the same healthy lifestyle changes.

MYTH: Children need kid-type foods because they have different tastes from adults.

WHY WE THINK THAT: Many of us have grown up being told by our doctors and our families that children have sensitive pallets and need bland, sweet, or special foods.

THE FACTS: Children are not born with sensitive taste buds that require coddling. They have the same taste buds as adults. As parents, we teach our children how to develop preferences for certain foods and how to learn to make choices. If a child is offered a wide variety of mostly whole foods, along with different ways to season the food, they will learn to like and seek out these types of foods. On the other hand, if children

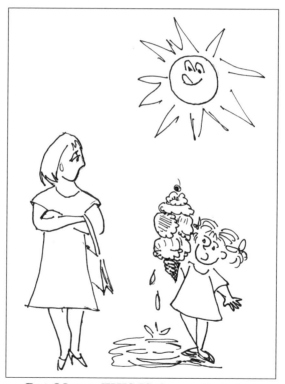

But, Mama, THIS IS the smallest size.

are given refined and processed foods or junk foods that are sweet, salty, bland, or fatty, then they will grow up with a taste for these foods.

We need to introduce our babies and children to different foods, tastes, and textures early. This will increase our children's desire for a variety of different types of foods

> *We need to introduce our babies and children to different foods, tastes, and textures early.*

and will introduce a wide range of vitamins and nutrients to our child's diet. This is a good way to start them off in life with positive, healthy eating habits.

MYTH: Parents just need to tell their children "no."

WHY WE THINK THAT: As parents, we are in control of our children's food choices. We make the money and we do the shopping.

THE FACTS: We do need to control what our children eat but it can be an uphill battle. Food companies target children with advertising using anything they can to over-ride parental authority — from toys and cartoon characters to directly marketing to children on their electronic devices and even their clothing. Advertisers know children are not mentally aware of being manipulated and they view parents as the enemy. Think about the types of foods children see advertised on TV and the types of foods placed on the grocery store shelves right at small children's eye level. Kelly Stitt, a senior branch manager for Heinz Ketchup Division says, "You want that nag factor so that seven-year-old Sarah is nagging mom in the grocery stores to buy Funky Purple. We're not sure mom would reach out for it on her own."

Children need parents to make healthy choices for them and not give in to all their demands. Food advertisers know that children will

> *If nothing else, a tantrum at least provides physical activity!*

wear parents down by nagging and throwing tantrums to get the refined, fatty, sugary foods they see advertised. Giving in to a child's tantrum only shows that tantrums are rewarded and the child is in charge. If nothing else, a tantrum at least provides physical activity! Think how different our children's preferences might be if the manufacturers of fresh fruits and vegetables, salmon, and chicken sponsored children's TV programs and movies and showed delicious meals in their ads. Instead, children see ads from manufacturers of fast foods, refined snacks, sugary drinks, and processed cereals.

The bottom line: WE are the parents so WE are responsible for our children's choices.

MYTH: Food additives and preservatives don't affect our children's behavior.

WHY WE THINK THAT: We trust the products we buy for our children. We only buy the best.

THE FACTS: Artificial colors and the food preservative, sodium benzoate, have been shown to increase hyperactivity in some children.[78] When foods that contain food additives are consumed on a daily basis, hyperactivity in children becomes more noticeable. The food

> *Artificial colors and the food preservative, sodium benzoate, have been shown to increase hyperactivity in some children.*

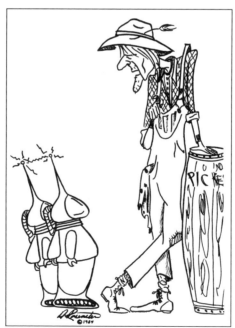

Boys, I don't give out samples to young 'uns without a Ma or Pa.

additives and artificial coloring don't make a child a raving, crazed monster, but their normal activity levels are temporarily and noticeably altered. They might take longer to settle down for a nap, or not sit as quietly when first asked to do so, or not pay attention as closely when spoken to until the food moves through their system. A greater concern is that we may be feeding our children foods that do more than nourish them.

What to take away

- Children don't need special "kid" foods.
- We adults are responsible for teaching our children good, healthy eating habits.
- What a nursing mother eats enters her milk and affects her baby.

24. DETOXIFYING

I've been on a diet for two weeks and all I've lost is two weeks.
— Totie Fields

Some of us believe that the way to lose weight and become healthy is to ingest different types of pills, avoid certain foods, or drink a mixture of fruit and vegetable juices, sometimes laced with laxatives. We even flood our colons with copious amounts of water or other liquids in an effort to purge our bodies of perceived toxins, chemicals, and excess fats. A lot of us purchase detoxification (detox) aids looking for a miracle to lose weight, prevent disease, eliminate cellulite, rejuvenate the skin, reduce bloating, and cleanse the body of material supposedly impacted in the colon. The truth is that there is no evidence to support any of these claims.

The theory behind a detox diet is that our bodies are continually bombarded with toxins, which build up in our system and cause problems. Detoxing has become a multi-million dollar industry, with products and supplements to help expel these so-called unwanted toxins while promising miraculous results. Promoting dietary change is at the core of most of the detox diets. The foods allowed and not allowed can vary widely, but generally fruit, vegetables, beans, nuts, seeds, herbal teas, and massive amounts of water are allowed. In contrast, wheat, dairy, meat, fish, eggs, caffeine, alcohol, salt, sugar, and processed foods are banned. Of course, these are the foods most people love and some of them contain necessary nutrients.

Detox diets are marketing myths rather than nutritional reality. "Detox is a meaningless term that is used all the time and because it hasn't been defined, it's impossible to say if it has worked or if it hasn't," says a spokesman for the British Dietetic Association.[79]

> Detox diets are marketing myths rather than nutritional reality.

The easiest way to prevent disease and lose unwanted weight is simply a change in diet and a workable exercise program. Our body's organs are designed to extract nutrition from food and eliminate waste material without any help from branded pills, enemas, or juices! Archeologists have been unearthing the remnants of bodies for years, and these bodies don't have impacted colons.

"The detox fad or fads, as there are many methods, is an example of the capacity of people to believe in and pay for magic despite the lack of any sound evidence," says Martin Wiseman, professor of human nutrition at the University of Southampton.[80]

Most of the pills, juices, teas, and oils that are sold for their detoxifying effects have no scientific foundation for their claims, according to Wiseman. Drinking tap water, eating a balanced diet, exer-

> *Most of the pills, juices, teas, and oils that are sold for their detoxifying effects have no scientific foundation for their claims.*

cising, and getting a good night's sleep will have the same effect. A recent study by American researchers concluded that detox diets do no more than the body's own natural system to get rid of toxins. They said most modern books and detox kits serve up "empty promises." Scientists and dieticians argue that the benefits people feel are not due to their body getting rid of excessive toxins but are due to improving what was likely a "poor" diet.

We tend to forget that the body is equipped with a detoxification system of its own, which includes the following:

- The skin. The main function of the body's largest organ is to provide a barrier against harmful substances, bacteria, viruses, heavy metals, and chemical toxins. The skin is a one-way defense system. Toxins are not eliminated through sweat and perspiration.
- The respiratory system. Fine hairs inside the nose trap dirt and other large particles that may be inhaled. Smaller particles that make it to the lungs are expelled from the airways in mucus.
- The immune system. This network of cells and molecules is designed to recognize foreign substances and eliminate them from the body.

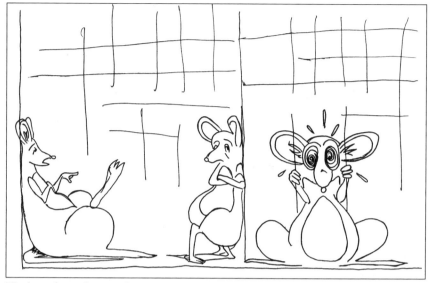

He just found out what a colonic detox really is.

- The intestines. Peyer's patches are lymph nodes in the small intestine that screen out parasites and other foreign substances before nutrients are absorbed into the blood from the colon.

- The liver. The liver is the body's principal filter, and produces a family of proteins called metallothioneins, which are also found in the kidneys. Metallothioneins not only metabolize food but also neutralize harmful metals like lead, cadmium, and mercury to prepare for their elimination from the body. Liver cells also produce groups of enzymes that regulate the metabolism of drugs and are an important part of the body's defense against harmful chemicals and other toxins.

- The kidneys. Urine tests are used to screen for drugs and toxins. This shows that the kidneys are very effective in filtering waste substances and moving them out of the body.[81]

Let's look at the myths of detox aids:

MYTH: Our bodies are flooded with harmful chemicals and toxins that cause cancer and other diseases.

WHY WE THINK THAT: We are inundated with "studies" that tell us we are being bombarded with toxins from water, air, and food and that these toxins cause cancer.

THE FACTS: A chemical is any substance with a distinct molecular composition that is produced by, or used in, a chemical process. This means *everything* in the universe is made of chemicals, including our own bodies. Cancer is sometimes caused by chemicals that go awry in our bodies, but thousands of natural chemicals also cause cancer. Nicotine is the most prevalent. Hemlock is also a natural poison, as are arsenic and cyanide. Another natural substance, acrylamide, which is found in the non-bromated, unbleached flour used in "organic" breads, has produced tumors in laboratory rats.

"The dose makes the poison," as toxicologists say. Many chemicals that are dangerous in large doses are beneficial in smaller amounts. One is water and another is salt. Too much of either can be lethal. Too much vitamin A is toxic but, in the right dose, it is a necessary nutrient. Butylated hydroxytoluene (BHT) prevents baked goods and cereals from spoiling, and nitrates keep bacteria from growing in lunchmeats; both are vital to both economics and safety. Without them, we'd pay a lot more for food, and we would die of food poisoning more often.

Everything in the universe is made of chemicals, including our own bodies.

When manufacturers put additives in foods, they do so knowing the risks and benefits. I'm not saying the food supply is risk-free, because nothing can be risk-free. But the risks are well balanced, and that's one reason American longevity keeps rising. Life expectancy reached 77.9 years in 2004, and cancer deaths have been falling since 1990. Other nations have even better numbers because they have better diet and exercise patterns. The leading cause of death today is not cancer, its heart disease caused by smoking, obesity, and a lack of exercise.

MYTH: I need to take pills or liquids to detox my body.

WHY WE THINK THAT: Pills and liquids are easy to take and tend to work fast, and that makes us think we are "wiped clean."

THE FACTS: Most of the detox aids have no scientific foundation to back up their claims, and they aren't really necessary. The body's own detoxifiers, namely the liver, kidneys, skin, intestines, and lungs, are enough to remove and excrete toxins within hours of their consumption. Eating a diet of whole, unprocessed foods will ensure that these organs work to their full potential.

The best way to improve or "detox" our body is to make some simple, healthy changes in our diet. It isn't that our body has a build-up of crud, like a dirty gas filter from a car but, as with a car, the cleaner the fuel, the more efficiently the engine or body works.

> *The best way to improve or "detox" our body is to make some simple, healthy changes in our diet.*

If we simply drink more water, but not necessarily eight glasses a day, and eat more fruit and vegetables, our skin will look better and we will feel healthier. For example, one of the results of being fully hydrated and getting more natural antioxidants from fruits and veggies in our diet may be fewer headaches. Combine such results with removing from our diet what we know is bad for us like cigarettes, processed foods, and too much alcohol and we will compound that feeling of well-being.

Think about it: since our bodies have the capability to naturally detox, if we simply add foods we know are good for us, remove the ones we know are bad, and do more exercise, the body will take care of the rest.

MYTH: Dairy products and meats are full of toxins and fruits and vegetables are not.

WHY WE THINK THAT: We think of dairy and meat products as being "heavy" and fruit and vegetables as being "light," and we associate "light" with "clean."

THE FACTS: Detox diets often promote fruits and vegetables as being low in toxins while meat and fish are said to lead to the accumulation of harmful substances in the body. Dr. Rob Hicks, a writer for the

BBC's health website, says the opposite is often true. He says vegetables such as cabbage and onions are high in naturally occurring toxins, while meat and fish have low levels.[82] After all, Socrates drank hemlock tea to kill himself; he didn't eat beef stew! However, any food can spoil, accumulate toxic bacteria, or be contaminated by outside substances. Detoxing can actually be dangerous for groups such as teenagers or pregnant women, who should not deprive themselves of food from a variety of different groups.

MYTH: Detox diets are a safe way to lose weight.

WHY WE THINK THAT: Since detox methods can be bought over the counter without a doctor's recommendation, we think they are safe.

THE FACTS: Twenty-five-year-old Molly Davis lives a healthy lifestyle, but decided that she wanted to help her body "perform optimally."[83] She thought she needed to flush her system using the most popular detox regimen.

> *Detoxing can actually be dangerous for groups such as teenagers or pregnant women.*

For ten days, she didn't eat solid food, and she drank eight glasses or more a day of a concoction of lemon juice, water, maple syrup, and cayenne pepper. In the mornings, Molly drank two full quarts of salt water and in the evenings, she drank a laxative tea.

"I felt like hell," she said. Molly suffered from headaches, acne, and irritability, and a strange, whitish film covered her tongue. She lost ten pounds but, after stopping the diet, she regained the weight. Detox regimens are offered by hundreds of books and web sites. Spas and salons invite clients to spend thousands of dollars to starve themselves or follow strange diet regimens, sometimes in exotic locations.

Many dietitians and medical experts say these diets are pointless at best and dangerous at worst. Critics of detox regimens say that, like other fad diets, they promise quick weight loss that is ultimately unsustainable and is based on "junk science," rather than on a true understanding of how the body works to keep itself clean and healthy. Worst of all, extreme detox diets, like the one Molly followed, can cause serious side effects in certain people.

Detox diets give people a false sense of security and a feeling that they've been responsible about their health. When the diet is over, people go back to their normal way of eating. Many detox regimes use laxatives or excessive amounts of liquids that behave like a laxative. This raises red flags among dietitians because laxatives are commonly abused by people who have eating disorders, such as bulimia, because they believe laxatives are useful for weight control. Excessive laxative use can cause severe dehydration and heart and colon damage. Colonic irrigation, a process in which lots of liquid is forced into the colon through a tube, is another fixture of some detox diets. Irrigation carries the risk of bowel perforation or infection either of which can cause death.

MYTH: Detox is necessary to get healthy and stay healthy.

WHY WE THINK THAT: Just like we routinely deep clean our houses, we think we need to routinely deep clean our bodies from the inside out.

THE FACTS: Those who believe in detoxing say the body is under constant assault from toxins, such as smog, pesticides, artificial sweeteners, sugar, and alcohol. They say that, without a periodic cleansing, these poisons accumulate in the body and cause headaches, fatigue, and a variety of chronic diseases. But we know the body already has a system of multiple organs to keep us safe and clean. Furthermore, there is no real evidence that toxins from foods or the environment accumulate within the body to the point of causing a "drainage backup," nor do detox diets alter the way the body's own system works.

Most detox regimens urge dieters to consume basic items, such as water and raw fruits or vegetables. Some detox diets also recommend *Detox causes the body to eliminate valuable nutrients.* laxatives, enemas, or colonic irrigation to speed up the detox process. This really means we can't make any social plans because we need to stay close to the bathroom! This also causes the body to eliminate valuable nutrients because the body doesn't have enough time to absorb any of the nutrition taken in before elimination takes place. It's true that the average person doesn't always drink enough water or consume enough fruits and vegetables. But we can eat them and enjoy them without putting ourselves through the uncomfortable phases of a detox regimen. We don't need to worry about phantom toxins to the point of doing bodily damage in an effort to purge ourselves. The problem is that most detox diets are so restrictive that they're ineffective for long-term use. And any weight loss is likely to be temporary because fat is not lost; water is lost, and is soon gained back.

Those who believe in detox diets will report a variety of benefits, such as fewer headaches, clearer skin, and weight loss, but none can be clearly traced to the implementation of detoxification.

> *Most detox diets are so restrictive that they're ineffective for long-term use.*

Fewer headaches can be attributed to other healthier, permanent lifestyle changes such as reduction in consumption of nicotine, alcohol, caffeine, and processed food. Clearer skin can result from decreased sun exposure, reduction of nicotine, improved hydration, reduction in processed-food intake, and a switch to whole, natural foods. Less bloating can be a result of eating better foods, and less of them. Scientists and dieticians argue that the benefits people feel from detox are due to changing from what likely was a "poor" diet to an improved one rather than their body getting rid of excessive toxins that weren't there in the first place. Some people who use detox diets report a boost in energy and even a sense of euphoria. Note that these feelings are also reported by people who are fasting; they are the body's reaction to starvation and a natural way to help us evade threats and locate food.

The bottom line: Promoters of detox diets promise a quick fix and a healthy, slim body but, in fact, are selling another gimmick on the diet roulette wheel. A person can detox for ten days, or use those ten days to make the transition to a balanced diet with correct proportions of whole, unprocessed foods, coupled with exercise.

If we are eating foods that are harmful or toxic, a branded pill, juice, or enema won't save our liver from alcohol, our arteries from plaque, our lungs from smoke, or our body from excess weight. Branded detox aids feed on our desire for a quick fix. And like all quick fixes, if they sound too good to be true, they are exactly that. Cutting out unhealthy foods, eating naturally, and drinking adequate amounts of water will help our

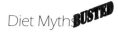
organs do what they were designed by Mother Nature to do. If our doctor thinks we really need to be cleaned out, we can drink a bottle of Fleet. This is what most doctors recommend just before a colonoscopy.

What to take away

- Detox diets are not necessary and are a gimmick.
- Detox diets can be dangerous and do not provide proper nutrition.
- Our bodies naturally detoxify themselves.

25. ORGANIC, CONVENTIONAL AND LOCAL FOODS

Old people shouldn't eat health foods. They need all the preservatives they can get.

— Robert Orben

At no point in human history has food been safer than it is today. Our modern agricultural methods have sanitized our food to the point where we can eat almost without fear. This is true for all food, organic and conventional. The issue for this chapter is the ongoing debate about which is really better, organically produced food or conventionally produced food, and the role local production plays in the debate.

Starting in the 20th century a vast array of new synthetic chemicals were introduced to the food growing process to increase supply, prevent crop and animal

> Which is really better, organically produced food or conventionally produced food

loss, and thus provide more food for more people at a lower cost. The questions that have come up look at whether these new practices are the best way to raise food. Are they healthy, safe for people and the environment, sustainable, and producing the most nutritious food? The answers to these questions are mixed and remain controversial.

These days "conventional" farms are the ones using the synthetic chemicals. Organic farms limit the use of synthetic chemicals, which somehow makes them "unconventional," even though the methods they use have been conventional since the dawn of agriculture. Even though they don't make a lot of sense, we will use the terms ("organic" and "conventional") that we are given.

Organic farms produce food in a way that limits the use of synthetic materials during production. For the vast majority of human history, agriculture can be described as organic as we use the term today. Until the twentieth century, farmers didn't have any synthetic chemical

233

weapons against fungus, bugs, and disease. Under organic production, the use of these non-organic pesticides, insecticides, and herbicides is greatly restricted and used only as a last resort. However, contrary to popular belief, certain non-organic fertilizers are still used.

Commercial organic food production is a heavily regulated industry that has been growing at an annual rate of 20 percent for the past couple of decades, and is now worth $23 billion in global sales.

> *Under organic production, the use of conventional non-organic pesticides, insecticides, and herbicides is greatly restricted*

The success of the organic food market has to do with the belief that not using synthetic pesticides and fertilizers makes food safer and more nutritious. Currently, the European Union, the United States, Canada, Japan, and many other countries require producers to obtain a special certification in order to market food as "organic" within their borders. Most certifications allow some chemicals and pesticides to be used, so consumers should be aware of the standards for qualifying as "organic" in their respective locales.

Organically raised livestock and poultry must be reared without the routine use of antibiotics or growth hormones and generally fed a healthy diet that meets the needs of their bodies. For example, cows are not fed corn since their digestive systems don't handle it well. Instead, they are grass fed. Animals from 100% local organic farms are allowed to live their lives naturally in free-range pastures, fields, and yards. In large organic stockyards the animals are fed well but they live in more crowded, structured conditions. Conventionally raised animals are free range and grass fed for only a small part of their lives. After that, they are crowded into pens at the stockyards and fed corn, antibiotics, and reprocessed feed.

Historically organic farms have been relatively small, family-run operations, which is why organic food was once only available in small stores or farmers' markets. Today this is what we would define as a sustainable source of food. The sustainable agricultural system is one that is considered ecologically sound, economically viable, and socially just. It is a system capable of maintaining productivity almost indefinitely. Sometimes, groups of neighboring farms pool their resources into a co-op and are able to sell larger quantities of food and more variety. They are sometimes financed by charging customers for not only the food but also a membership fee.

Industrialized agriculture has become "conventional" only within the last 60 or so years, since World War II. It is a multi-trillion-dollar industry worldwide. Conventional foods are from farms that are industrialized agricultural systems characterized by mechanization, monocultures, and the use of synthetic inputs such as chemical fertilizers and pesticides, with an emphasis on maximizing productivity and profitability. Conventional farming and increased ability to economically ship food from around the world has allowed all sorts of foods to become economical, abundant, and available all year round.

So which is better? A recent publication from the United Kingdom's Food Standards Agency (FSA) and published in the *American Journal of Clinical Nutrition* found that organically and conventionally produced foods are equal in their nutrient content. The study was based on a review of 55 relevant studies conducted over the past 50 years.[84]

Organically and conventionally produced foods are equal in their nutrient content.

Supporters of the study will reference numerous supporting conclusions reached over the past two decades and stress that the FSA report was the most comprehensive examination of organic health claims ever undertaken. Opponents will also reference numerous contrasting conclusions reached over the past two decades and note that the FSA report failed to measure antioxidants and pesticide residues. Those who support organic agriculture can cite a 2007 report from Newcastle University showing that organic produce has 40 percent more antioxidants than conventional produce.[85] Those who discount organics might refer to a 2000 study that found no effect on the levels of healthful phenols in organic strawberries and blueberries verses conventionally grown strawberries and blueberries.[86] Or perhaps they'd choose a report that found higher rates of naturally occurring toxins in organic foods on account of their being grown without the benefit of synthetic fungicides.[87] These studies are grounded in science, but what do they tell us, the consumer who's trying to decide what to buy and what to eat? Both sides have

Table 9: Conventional vs. Organic Farming

Conventional	Organic
Apply chemical fertilizers to promote plant growth.	Apply natural fertilizers, such as manure or compost, to feed soil and plants.
Spray insecticides to reduce pests and disease.	Use beneficial insects and birds, mating disruption, or traps to reduce pests and disease.
Use chemical herbicides to manage weeds.	Rotate crops, till, hand weed, or mulch to manage weeds.
Give animals antibiotics, growth hormones, and medications to prevent disease and spur growth.	Give animals organic feed and allow them access to the outdoors. Use preventive measures — such as rotational grazing, a balanced diet, and clean housing — to help minimize disease.

legitimate arguments and this is why consumers like you and me are confused and frustrated.

There are no broad public health issues at stake here. People aren't dying in large numbers or becoming supermen because they eat either conventional or organic foods. Organic food often costs more than conventional and comprises only 3.7% of the food eaten in the United States (11.4% of fruit and vegetables)[88], so most people still choose to eat conventional foods.

Another part of this food debate is the comparison between farming practices. The truth can be hard to find. I'm not going to get involved except to point out that both methods have their risks and both have their benefits. It all depends on the farmer using methods that make the particular form of farming safe. Table 9 summarizes the differences between conventional and organic farming.

One question that might be worth a quick note involves the yield of farms. Conventional farm supporters say that organic yields are about half the conventional yields. Organic supporters have studies that show comparable yields in America and higher yields for organic methods in poor countries.[89]

A more important issue in deciding where to get your food involves where it is grown. If you are looking for good nutrition, eat the freshest food possible. Food from your own garden, minutes after it is picked, is ideal. It works well to buy well-ripened food at a farmers' market if the food was harvested the day before. Buying food that was picked green, covered with wax to preserve appearance, flown halfway around the world, and left to sit in the produce aisle for a week is not going to get you the best-tasting or most nutritious food. The clear rule is, buy locally and in season, when you can. Out of season, frozen and canned food may be a better choice.

According to B. J. Friedman, a nutritionist at Texas State University — San Marcos, only one-quarter of Americans eat the recommended

> *If you are looking for good nutrition, eat the freshest food possible.*

five or more servings of fruits and vegetables each day. Instead of trying to prove one system is better than the other, we should focus on a more critical public health issue. The majority of our population is overweight and undernourished. Too many people don't eat a variety of whole unprocessed foods and the foods they do eat are nutritionally deficient. Worse, they are consumed in portions that are too large. Rather than worry about eating organic or conventional, we need to worry more about eating whole fresh, unprocessed foods, in a balanced and proportional manner.

So what do we eat? Don't think of food as being organic or conventional; think of food as being real or chemically enhanced. The easiest way to decide what to eat is to eat only what your great-grandmother

> *The easiest way to decide what to eat is to eat only what your great-grandmother would recognize as food.*

would recognize as food. That means you don't eat the numerous processed products, such as sugary cereals, processed candy bars, crackers, and phony cheese-like foodstuffs that outnumber real food and real cheese. Don't eat anything that is incapable of rotting. Foods that have chemically altered fats and fillers have a long shelf life and don't break down, and they will also not break down easily in your body. Avoid food products containing ingredients that are unfamiliar, unpronounceable,

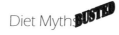

and that include high-fructose corn syrup (HFCS) or hydrogenated fats. Avoid foods packaged with a health claim because these are processed foods with added nutrients rather than whole foods. It's easier to put a health-claim sticker on a box of sugary cereal than on a head of cabbage or a blueberry. The healthiest foods in the supermarket are usually found in the produce section and in the dairy and meat cases along the outside perimeter of the grocery store.

Now for the myths:

MYTH: Large, commercially run organic farms always practice organic techniques so the food they sell to the large supermarket chains is really organic.

WHY WE THINK THAT: We want to trust what is sold as organic from our favorite supermarket and we want the best value for our money.

THE FACTS: The organic food business is a multi-billion dollar business. Producing high volumes of produce and animal products

The organic food business is a multi-billion dollar business.

unconventionally is costly, time consuming and often impractical. In order to compete with conventionally grown products, pure organic practices are often compromised. In 2002, the federal government created the National Organic Rule. According to Congress, organic food is food or products produced without synthetic fertilizers, conventional pesticides, growth hormones, genetic engineering, or germ-killing radiation. However, there are varying levels of "organic-ness."

Some products are made with both organic and conventional ingredients, which means the food is at least 70% organic. They are labeled as "Made with organic ingredients." What isn't stated is not all the ingredients are organic. The government defines foods that are organic as anything made with 90% organic ingredients. Even though the food may be made with organic ingredients, they are not necessarily all grown using strict organic farming methods. If it says 100% organic, then the products are made exclusively with all organic ingredients and were grown using organic farming methods.[90]

Even if you buy organic food from large food chains, the freshness may be compromised due to how far and how long the food item has traveled. Once the produce is picked, it starts to lose its nutrient value regardless of whether it is conventional or organic.

If you want a guarantee that what you purchase and consume is 100% organic and fresh, buy from *Buy locally for the best food.*

sustainable local farms, orchards, and ranches or farmers markets and local fresh meat markets. The government defines sustainable farms as an integrated system of plant and animal production practices having a site-specific application that will, over the long term, satisfy human food and fiber needs; enhance environmental quality and the natural resource base upon which the agricultural economy depends; make the most efficient use of nonrenewable resources and on-farm resources, and integrate, where appropriate, natural biological cycles and controls; sustain the economic viability of farm operations; and enhance the quality of life for farmers and society as a whole. All the food is raised locally and travels minimally so the items are always fresh.[91]

MYTH: Organic fruits and vegetables have more nutrition than conventional fruits and vegetables.

WHY WE THINK THAT: Since organic food is farmed without conventional chemicals in soil that has been specially cultivated and cared for, the food should be of better quality.

THE FACTS: This is both true and false. The time the food has been on the shelf and the amount of time the food has spent traveling to the market affect the level of nutrition more than the soil or fertilizer used to grow it. For example, in Minnesota where my family lives, apples are in season in September and October. A number of large, commercially run, conventional orchards in Minnesota bombard the supermarkets with a variety of apples at that time. Even though the orchards are commercial and use chemicals to ensure a good harvest, the apples are still locally produced. Other apples that are organic but from Washington state are also available. Since the apples from Washington have traveled a further distance for a longer period of time, their organic nutrition has had more time to erode away than the conventionally grown, local apples.

On the other hand, my husband and I know a couple who have a small apple orchard that they tend themselves without using chemicals.

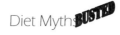

Every fall they invite us and other friends over to harvest as many apples as we want straight off the tree. The ones we eat right after they have been picked will have the most nutrients. Fruits and vegetables that are flash frozen right after picking also retain their nutrition better than those that sit out for days on display.

MYTH: Organic meat and conventional meat are the same.

WHY WE THINK THAT: Meat is meat, no matter where it comes from. Plus our country has very high standards for meat.

THE FACTS: When it comes to meat, organic may actually be better but only by a small degree. Both organic and conventional meats must meet the same USDA safety standards.

Both organic and conventional meats must meet the same USDA safety standards.

However, the meats are generated by different means. Animals, such as chickens, cows, and pigs, grown conventionally for meat are fed the by-products of mammalian or poultry slaughter. The FDA banned the feeding of cattle brains and spinal tissue in 1997, and recently banned the feeding of blood, blood products, human food waste, and poultry litter. However, the FDA still allows cattle to be fed gelatin rendered from the hooves of cattle and other species; fats, oils, grease, tallow from cattle and other species; poultry and poultry by-products, rendered pork protein, and rendered horse protein.

Animals raised on an organic farm are fed grass, not grain. Animals raised for organic meat can't have any animal by-products in their feed, primarily because some animal byproducts are associated with mad-cow disease. They are allowed to roam, so their meat is lower in fat, are not injected with hormones, and are not fed large amounts of antibiotics. Grazing animals were meant to graze on grasses. Grass-fed beef contains higher amounts of omega-3 fatty acids, which are in short supply in the American diet, compared to corn-fed beef.

Conventionally raised animals are fed a feed made of animal parts and grains to fatten them up before they go to the stockyards. The animals are given antibiotics to counter problems they have because their systems are not able to effectively process grain. Any medications and hormones given to the animals tend to be stored in the fat and not in the muscle tissue. Conventional meat that comes from animals that are fed a corn-based diet puts more fat on the animal, and the type of fat is omega-6. The American diet is overloaded with omega-6: we eat corn, we eat breads and pasta made with corn, we fry our foods in corn oil, and we feed our meat sources corn.

If you wish to purchase conventionally produced meats, don't consume the fat, since it may contain residual drugs or hormones. However, a well-fed animal is going to produce a better, higher-quality meat.

Organic meat is about the most expensive organic food item you can purchase. Organic ground beef can cost as much as seven dollars a pound while conventional ground

> *A well-fed animal is going to produce a better, higher-quality meat.*

beef may cost less than two dollars a pound. Since the fat of the animal is where the toxins are stored, a good compromise might be to buy conventional meat in the form of steaks or roasts but buy organic when it comes to ground meat and sausage, since the fat is mixed in with the muscle in ground meats.

A better way to get meat at a better price is to buy it locally from an organic farm and even have it butchered on site. Many local organic farms sell sides of beef and pork, and this larger quantity tends to be cheaper per pound. Another advantage to organic meats, such as sausage, is that nitric oxidizers are not used as preservatives, especially if the product is made on site.

Our family buys meats that are from locally owned farms, commercially organic and also conventionally processed. We buy chicken that is commercially organic in that the chicken has not been given antibiotics or growth hormones, however they are not necessarily free range. The price is competitive to the standard conventionally processed chicken. We buy conventional beef, pork, and lamb in the form of steaks and roasts but buy ground meat and ground turkey from local organic markets. We buy breakfast sausage, both pork and turkey, from a store that makes their own from meat purchased from local farms. This is because conventional prepackaged sausage or other breakfast meat is preserved with nitrates. This is one way we compromise between eating organic and being economical.

MYTH: You don't have to be as careful about washing organic food.

WHY WE THINK THAT: We believe that since natural methods of growing organic foods are practiced, there are no chemical residues on the produce.

THE FACTS: Whether organic or conventional, we need to rinse off our produce to remove the dust and dirt that accumulates from

Whether organic or conventional, we need to rinse off our produce.

being handled and sitting on the grocery-store shelves. As for concern about pesticide residues on conventional foods, the daily dose received by average consumers is at least several thousand times below the level that government experts consider safe. Faced with mounting government concern, manufacturers of the organic pesticide, rotenone, have decided to stop selling it for use on cranberries, cereal grains, and harvested tomatoes. Ongoing research has found a replacement, spinosad, which may be used by both organic and conventional growers. It appears to be effective on many harmful insects while not significantly affecting beneficial insects.

Here is a list of the foods that may be better to buy organic if you are more comfortable knowing they were grown without chemical protection:

- Apples
- Cherries
- Grapes
- Nectarines

- Peaches
- Pears
- Raspberries
- Strawberries

- Bell peppers
- Celery
- Potatoes
- Spinach

Foods that are fine to buy conventional:

- Pineapple
- Kiwi
- Banana
- Mango
- Papaya
- Blueberries

- Watermelon
- Melons
- Onions
- Avocado
- Sweet corn
- Sweet peas

- Asparagus
- Cabbage
- Broccoli
- Eggplant

MYTH: All organic food is better.

WHY WE THINK THAT: Since we believe organic food is free of chemicals and additives, thus in its natural state, we assume it is better quality.

THE FACTS: Not if it's organic chips, organic soda, or organic cookies. No matter what kind of compost was or wasn't used to nurture the potatoes, or how pure the sugar is, fried chips are still fried and cane sugar is still sugar. Too many non-essential calories, whether from organic ingredients or conventional ingredients, will still be stored as fat.

The benefits of organic foods and their superiority over foods grown under conventional methods have been extolled by people for a long time, but there is substantial evidence that organic foods do not offer special culinary, health, or safety benefits.

Fried chips are still fried and cane sugar is still sugar.

A recent poll shows that 67% of consumers think USDA-certified organic foods are superior to conventional foods.[92] However, blind taste-tests consistently show that people cannot distinguish between organic

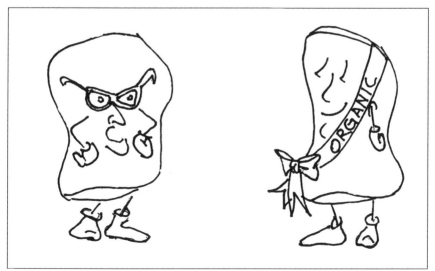

I don't care if you're organic, you're still just a deep-fried potato chip like me.

and conventional foods and, when the labels are switched, consumers often prefer the phony "organic" products![93]

Research confirms that organic and conventional foods almost always have the same nutritional value. Studies keep flip-flopping on this. One study found more vitamin C in organic tomatoes than in conventional ones.[94] Another found more cancer-fighting flavonoids in organic corn and strawberries.[95] However, other studies haven't found organics to have a nutritional edge.

The bottom line: What makes the biggest difference in nutrient content is how long produce sits on the shelf. Fresh spinach, for instance, loses about half of its folic acid, a B vitamin, within a week, whether it is conventional or organic.[96]

MYTH: Organic food tastes better.

WHY WE THINK THAT: We have been led to believe that organic is a purer form of food and therefore will taste better, and many of us can swear to that.

THE FACTS: Nobody has been able to tell the difference between commercial conventional and commercial organic foods, except in one study involving apples where organics came out ahead. To get

Nothing is at its best when it's waxed, flown halfway around the world, and spends weeks in the grocery store.

raspberries that taste "raspberrier," and blueberries that taste "bluer" buy produce that's locally grown, in season, and hasn't been sitting on the shelf too long, or visit any of the "you-pick-it-yourself" farms for seasonal produce. Nothing is at its best when it's waxed, flown halfway around the world, and spends weeks in the grocery store.

MYTH: Organic food is expensive.

WHY WE THINK THAT: Just go to any organic grocery store and look at the prices.

THE FACTS: For some food items this statement is true, but for others it is not. Conventional food prices don't reflect hidden costs borne by taxpayers. Hidden costs may include federal subsidies and pesticide regulation and testing.

Most people who choose to eat organic food either grow it themselves, buy it locally (from a co-op, health food store, or farmer's market), buy directly (from a distribution warehouse or a food buying club), join a community-supported agriculture program (buy directly from a local farmer), or go to a U-Pick farm (where you pick your own and pay per pound). All of these avoid charges associated with transportation and the storage of food. When organic food from local farms, orchards, or farmers markets are bought in season, this can balance out the effects of the less nutritious nature of some large supermarket organic food production due to time spent traveling and sitting on a shelf.

Discount super chains such as Wal-Mart, the country's number-one seller of organic milk, are slashing the organic markup to 10% while at most places the mark-up is 20%-30%. Organics aren't just for the elite anymore.

Organics aren't just for the elite anymore.

MYTH: Organic food is 100% pesticide-free.

WHY WE THINK THAT: We think of pesticides as chemicals, we have been cautioned against ingesting them, and we believe that chemicals are not used on organic crops.

THE FACTS: While organic farmers don't apply synthetic chemicals to crops, they are permitted to use organic pesticides. The organic designation never meant 100% pesticide- or chemical-free, despite public perception. The designation actually describes a method of farming that is as free of man-made chemicals as it can be. Synthetic pesticides are now so widespread that they appear regularly in the rainwater that drenches all crops, conventional and organic alike. These chemicals can also drift through the air, from conventional fields onto organic fields located miles away.

MYTH: If we eat organic foods, we are supporting small local farms and co-ops.

WHY WE THINK THAT: Since many of the organic foods come from small farms and co-ops, we assume they are the major suppliers.

THE FACTS: Organic farming is big business. Although the organic movement has humble origins, today most organic food isn't produced on family farms in quaint villages or on hippie communes in Vermont or California. Instead, the industry has become dominated by the large corporations that, in the minds of many organic consumers, used to be villains. A single company currently controls about 70% of the market for organic milk. California grows about $400 million a year of organic produce, and half of it comes from just five farms.[97] The Organic Trade Association's membership list includes the biggest names in agribusiness: Archer Daniels Midland, Gerber, and Heinz.

General Mills owns the Cascadian Farms brand, Kraft owns Back to Nature and Boca Burger, and Kellogg's owns Morningstar Farms just to name a few. The demand for organic food is so high that these giant companies are importing organic ingredients as cheaply as possible from other countries. Whole Foods sold roughly $1 billion in produce last year, but only about 16% was locally grown.[98] When we buy locally from the farmers market or from sustainable farms, we are indeed getting high quality organic food and supporting our local growers at the same time.

Organic farming is big business.

The bottom line: There continues to be a debate about which is better, organic or conventional, and a lot of the debate has to do with politics, economics, and other beliefs that go outside the nutritional value of the food. It is hard to keep them separate. It is always best to chose whole and unprocessed foods over refined and processed foods whether conventionally produced or organically produced. Certain types of foods may be better when purchased as organic or from local co-ops and farmers markets and with other foods it is just personal preference. Consumers need to know that if they choose the right conventionally grown foods or organic foods, they will be meeting their nutritional needs.

What to take away

- Eat the meat and avoid the fat if you are worried about what the animal was fed.

- Whether organic foods taste better than conventional foods is a matter of individual taste. What matters more are the varieties that are consumed and the freshness of the product.
- There are pros and cons to organic and conventional foods so select carefully and do what is best for you and your family both nutritionally and economically.
- Consuming too much of any food, conventional or organic, will make us fat.

26. THE FOOD INDUSTRIES

An average of two rodent hairs per one hundred grams of peanut butter is allowed.
— FDA Government Guideline No. 20

Green clovers. Blue diamonds. Orange stars. Pink hearts. Purple horseshoes. Man, I never know if I'm looking at a bowl of cereal or having another acid flashback.
— Dave Henry

We have more food per person in the United States than in any other country in the world. The food industries produce close to 4,000 calories per person per day, twice the calories the average adult male needs daily. Food corporations have one primary mission: to sell food and beverages to consumers. It is in the food industries' best interest to have an over-weight, nutritionally uneducated, hungry population. Food companies sell food based on what will sell, not on what is healthy. If a food is in demand and it is also healthy, then the food companies will sell it, but if a food is healthy but not in high demand, the food companies will not go to any great lengths to make it available. It is interesting to note that Thomas Jefferson had the foresight to claim; "If people let government decide what foods they eat and what medicines they take, their bodies will soon be in as sorry a state as are the souls of those who live under tyranny."

Recent examples of food companies selling foods that are in demand as well as healthier are foods without trans fats. That is because the public has become more *Food companies sell food based on what will sell, not on what is healthy.* knowledgeable about the dangers of trans fats and has demanded foods without them. However, this is more of an exception than a rule. Food corporations want to keep us in the dark about what is in our foods. If we are to make informed food choices in an effort to improve our diets, then we need to understand just what is on our grocery store shelves.

The ingredients listed on food labels are not all the ingredients in the food item. Often, cancer-causing chemicals, such as acrylamides, are formed during high-heat processing, but it is not required that these be listed on the label. Monosodium glutamate (MSG) is hidden in foods under different names: yeast extract, torula yeast, hydrolyzed vegetable protein, and autolyzed yeast. These ingredients are used to enhance the taste of food, and are found in almost all vegetarian foods. The problem with MSG is that it can disrupt our appetite regulation and cause us to eat more food, which helps food companies increase their business. MSG can cause disruptions in our endocrine system, thus causing imbalances in our hormone production.

Makers of junk food spend billions of dollars marketing unhealthy foods to children. They use celebrities, cartoon characters, free gifts, and contests to entice children to eat

Makers of junk food spend billions of dollars marketing unhealthy foods to children.

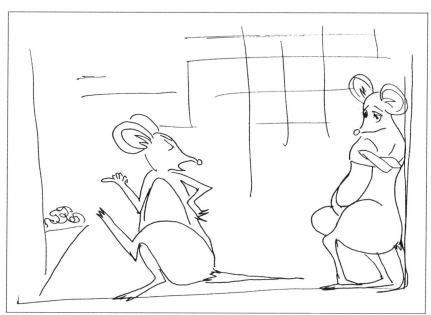

I'm not eating that stuff, it will give ya cancer.

their products. Junk-food manufacturers donate large sums of money to professional nutrition associations to legitimize their claims of health and nutrition in their foods. For example, the American Dietetic Association accepts money from Coca-Cola. We have an association devoted to curing diabetes, knowing the dangers of excess weight and a high sugar diet accepting money from a major manufacturer of a high-sugar drink.[99]

When food corporations take whole, unrefined foods and process them to meet or create demand, they are able to generate more profits from selling such foods, even though the food is now less healthy. These companies disguise their intentions and products by saying they sell healthy foods, but they're really not good for us. For example, major beverage makers agreed to remove sodas from school cafeterias and replaced them with juice drinks and sport drinks. Juice drinks and sport drinks have just as much or more added sugar as the sodas that were removed. In other words, no real change.

It is important to understand that the food industry uses their products to increase their business and ensure repeat business and they will do whatever it takes to make that happen. Profits come first, avoiding lawsuits next, and our health last.

> *It is important to understand that the food industry uses their products to increase their business and ensure repeat business.*

What to take away

- There is more in processed food than what is stated on the label.
- Food corporations have one fundamental mission: sell products.
- Chemicals in processed foods often interfere with and can be detrimental to our health.

27. GOOD FOODS GONE BAD

Ingredients as fresh as they were 27 years ago.
— Slogan of the Biscuitville restaurant

I think they should put a warning label on strawberries: "Caution: tastes nothing like a strawberry milkshake."
— Ryan Kaplan

We are told to eat more fish and add more fruits and vegetables to our diet. So we try to do just that. The food companies know this and do what they can to help us out. Or do they? Here are some examples:

Fish sticks. While made of fish, which contains omega-3, these are deep-fried in oil, thus changing good oils to hydrogenated oils (trans fats) that are known to cause health problems. The fish in fish sticks is usually pollock, which is a healthy fish. The breading that encases the fish is made of the remaining dozens of ingredients listed on the box, which aren't so healthy. Doctors and nutritionists have been advising us to eat more fish for years, because fish provide us with healthy fats and protein. Yet, when we consume processed fish products or when we order deep-fried fish from a fast-food restaurant, the refined and chemically altered ingredients overwhelm the good nutrition that was in the fish.

Yogurt. Essentially milk fermented with certain bacteria, yogurt is high in protein, calcium, and vitamins and can be eaten by anyone, especially adults who generally cannot easily digest milk.

Homemade yogurt is pure and uncomplicated.

Homemade yogurt is pure and uncomplicated. What is sold in many mainstream U.S. supermarkets as yogurt is closer to a dairy dessert loaded with sugar and processed fruit. Since it is sold as yogurt we believe it is a health food. A better choice is plain yogurt and our own fruit.

Soup. Healthy, inexpensive, and easy to make, a meal of homemade soup and whole-grain bread is fortified with wholesome nutrition. When a week's worth of homemade soup is prepared in bulk and frozen in individual containers, it costs less than a dollar a day. Canned soup is a concoction of salt, fat, artificial additives, preservatives, and water, with small amounts of vegetables and a bit of meat. One serving typically contains 1,000 milligrams of sodium, which is about half of our daily allowance. Soup is easy to make and it is inexpensive. Just save turkey, chicken, and beef bones and boil them for a stock. Then add vegetables and noodles along with herbs and spices to taste. Matzo balls or dumplings also add a nice touch. Make a couple of gallons and freeze some for future use.

Green tea. This beverage is widely consumed throughout Asia and has been elevated to an art form in Japan. Clinical studies have shown that all tea contains antioxidants and other healthful components that reduce the risks of cancer, heart disease, senility, and other diseases associated with aging. Most Americans don't appreciate the taste of tea so we buy what is often called "chai tea," which is loaded with sugar and other additives, then sold as a health drink. Any ingredients listed after the words "green tea" on the bottle generally destroys the health benefits of the tea.

Fruit juice. Fresh-squeezed juice is a nice alternative to eating whole fruit. The food industries have given us drinks that advertise that they are "made with real fruit

Fresh-squeezed juice is a nice alternative to eating whole fruit, especially if it contains the pulp.

juice." The packaging for some fruit drinks brags about being fortified with essential vitamins and minerals. So what is the rest of the drink? Sugar and water. Even 100% fresh-squeezed juice is a sugar bomb for our bodies. When juice is consumed as part of a meal of protein and fat, the effects of the sugar are diminished. We give our children fruit juice as a "healthy" alternative to soda. While the juice may indeed provide a small amount of nutrition, it still blasts our system with sugar.

Food companies often push fruit drinks as an alternative medicine. Some of these juices are noni juice, pomegranate juice, açai juice, and goji berry juice. As mentioned earlier, my nephew was recently diagnosed with type II diabetes. His mother told the family that he was going on a regimen of drinking goji berry juice, believing it would boost his immune system and lower his high blood sugar. Like many of these alternative-medicine juices, the juice of the featured berry or fruit is blended with more palatable fruit extracts and sweeteners, so the benefits of the miracle berries are diluted. A study demonstrated that when two groups of people were given either goji berry juice or a placebo, the health benefits for both groups were the same. Compared to conventional juices, goji berry juice didn't provide any additional health benefits and offered no improvement in blood sugar levels.

Any fruit juice will be viewed by my nephew's digestive system and ours as sugar, period. Regardless of how fantastic the supposed health claims may be, his blood sugar will rise and his insulin will spike. Adding sugar, whether under the guise of "medicine" or as a miracle cure, to the diet of a diabetic in an effort to control the disease is counterproductive.

Potatoes. Among the different varieties of potatoes, russets, with brown skin and white flesh, are only marginally healthy to begin with. They are cheap and hardy with few nutrients, and serve mostly as filler. The starch is quickly converted by the body into sugar, and too many servings may increase the risk of diabetes and obesity. They are the least flavorful and the cheapest of the hundreds of potato varieties available to us, so we do things to make them tasty. We cut them into strips, deep-fry them, and cover them with salt. Food companies dehydrate them, refine them, and put them in a box or bag, so all we have to do is add water.

Instead, we need to try different types of potatoes and consume all of them in the most whole and natural state possible. There are golden, red, and purple potatoes, just to name a few. These tend to have more nutrients than the russet variety.

> *We need to try different types of potatoes and consume all of them in the most whole and natural state possible.*

Popcorn. Today it barely resembles the healthy treat it used to be. Popcorn is high in fiber and low in calories, but that changes immensely when we or the movie theaters drown it in sugar, salt, and fat. Microwave popcorns are the biggest offenders because they have a long list of ingredients added to enhance the flavor. Buy popcorn kernels in bulk for pennies a serving, and use salt and real butter sparingly.

Bread. In the United States the most common form of bread is mass-produced, white, soft, and doughy with a shelf life of weeks, relatively cheap and abundant, and sold in plastic bags. Overconsumption of this type of bread is one major reason why we have so much obe-

> *Homemade bread is made of flour and water with a pinch of salt and some yeast, maybe along with an egg or two.*

sity and diabetes among our population. Homemade bread is made of flour and water with a pinch of salt and some yeast, maybe along with an egg or two. Packaged white bread contains dozens of other ingredients, such as sugar, corn syrup, hydrogenated oils, and preservatives. The natural nutrition has been removed and chemically reinstated. This processing creates a food product that, once eaten, is quickly converted to sugars that spike the blood sugar in our system. This causes the pancreas to work overtime to secrete insulin. Even mass-produced whole-wheat breads are unhealthy because they are made from refined wheat flour and an unhealthy combination of sugar, salt, and softening additives, along with lots of other ingredients.

Grains and cereals. Real grains and cereals, such as wheat, barley, rice, and rolled oats, are, and always have been, the human race's most important and basic food since we became an agricultural society. They offer an unbeatable combination of protein, healthy fat, and vitamins. Food producers have taken the word "cereal" and used it to describe tiny, crunchy, breakfast flakes or bits that are mixed or coated with sugar, corn syrup, salt, food dyes, and preservatives. Instead, eat far healthier and cheaper cereals such as rolled oats, rice, barley, or wheat in the form of meal or whole-grain with raisins, nuts, or fruit.

Organic food. The concept of organic food started out as a brilliant idea. Dedicated farmers would become stewards of the land and avoid using toxic chemical pesticides and fertilizers that had proliferated after World War II. They would raise food naturally and cultivate diverse crop varieties native to their soils. Animals raised for food would be treated with care and dignity. For thirty-some years, this was the case.

However, organic food has become so popular that its original value-system has become jeopardized. Big food entrepreneurs like Wal-Mart and Kraft want their share of the profits. To keep costs down and profits high, their demand for cheaper production methods undermines what it means to be organic. We can now buy organic milk from large farms on which hundreds of caged cows are fed organic grain but are still housed in crowded barns. We have organic junk food, with organic ingredients flown in from around the globe, disguised as health food by virtue of the "organic" label. Oreo-style cookies made with organic hydrogenated oil and organic refined sugars deliver the same non-nutritious number of calories as non-organic Oreo cookies. They just cost more. Organic potato chips aren't healthier than non-organic potato chips. Potato chips are potato chips.

Pizza. In Italy there are laws and specifications that define pizza. There are set rules concerning the type of flour, tomato, mozzarella, olive oil, basil, and oregano used. Pizza made this way is nutritious and filling. When our daughter went to Italy and had the pizza there, she was pleasantly surprised that it was made with fresh ingredients on the spot with a very thin crust. Most Americans have never eaten real pizza like this, and confuse it with the typical junk-food pizza advertised on American television, delivered to our homes, or sold in the grocery stores. When the Italians immigrated to the United States, street-corner pizza shops in Philadelphia, New York, and other large cities stuck to the original idea of simple, fresh ingredients. Then came the pizza chains, and they put most of those local shops out of business. Fresh ingredients were replaced with preservative-laden, cheap, and fatty ingredients for pizza that could be mass-produced, frozen, and shipped across the country. Commercial pizza is now a high-calorie, high-fat, high-sodium, low-nutrient food.

What to take away

- Real food does not need to contain added, unnecessary, refined ingredients.
- Food companies are generally more interested in profits than healthy eating.
- Homemade food is often cheaper and healthier.

28. Supplements

All those vitamins aren't to keep death at bay, they're to keep deterioration at bay.

— Jeanne Moreau

The supplement industry makes $15 billion a year from promoting and selling their pills and powders to 150 million Americans. Many of us take vitamins and mineral supplements, thinking we are enhancing our health without really understanding whether we truly need these extra vitamins. Many advertisers tell us that our fast-paced lifestyles prevent us from getting adequate vitamins and nutrients because we consume foods that are convenient rather than nutritious. These advertisers encourage us to take a pill or mix a powder with water to make up for our lack of nutrition.

The best way to get enough vitamins and minerals into our diet is to consume them in the form of whole, natural foods. Unprocessed, unrefined foods contain all the vitamins, minerals, fiber, and phyto-

> *The best way to get enough vitamins and minerals into our diet is to consume them in the form of whole, natural foods.*

chemicals we need for optimum health. No evidence supports the notion that taking vitamins and supplements is a better choice than consuming a well-balanced, healthy diet. However, many of us don't have the perfect diet, so supplements can help to fill in the gaps. Notice that we are talking about adding supplements to our diet, not substitutes for good, wholesome meals.

Studies show that most of us don't follow the dietary guidelines. These guidelines suggest that we should try to eat four or five servings of fruits and vegetables a day. To get the recommended calcium requirement, we need the equivalent of four glasses of milk. For the recommended amount of daily protein, we need the equivalent of a can of salmon with bones. For the recommended amount of fiber, we would need two cups of black-bean soup or all those servings of fruits and vegetables. Since these recommendations are not fully followed, the most common vitamins lacking in our diets are A, C, D, and E. The most common minerals that are lacking are calcium, magnesium, potassium and most diets lack fiber.

If we choose to take supplements, it is best to get them from sources that use natural ingredients instead of synthetic ingredients. We should also consult our physician to be sure we need them and that they don't interfere with any medications we might be taking.

MYTH: Men and women need the same supplements.

WHY WE THINK THAT: Everyone needs the same basic nutrition so one multivitamin should do it.

THE FACTS: A multivitamin is a good choice for most people, but our age and sex do play a role in what we need. Women need folic

A multivitamin is a good choice for most people.

acid to prevent birth defects. Since half of pregnancies are unplanned, women of childbearing age should have 400 micrograms of folic acid daily, just to be safe. Our hormones change as we age, and can affect our requirement for different vitamins and minerals, so men and women may need different types and amounts of certain vitamins at various ages. What we need is best determined by a physical check-up by our primary-care physician. As both men and women age, they may not absorb adequate amounts of B_{12} and vitamin D.

MYTH: A multivitamin is all we need.

WHY WE THINK THAT: They do contain everything.

THE FACTS: Almost true. A multivitamin is all most of us really need. Look for a vitamin that has 100% of the RDA and makes adjustments for gender and age. Multivitamins don't always contain more specialized supplements, such as fish oil, calcium, and magnesium. They should not cost a lot.

MYTH: No matter where we live, all vitamin dosages are the same.

WHY WE THINK THAT: We are all alike, so geography shouldn't matter.

THE FACTS: Those of us who live in the northern half of the northern hemisphere or the southern half of the southern hemisphere need extra doses of vitamin D. When our skin is exposed to sunlight, our bodies make vitamin D. However, during the fall and winter in those parts of the hemispheres, there isn't enough sunlight for our bodies to generate adequate amounts of vitamin D. Low levels of vitamin D are associated with gum disease, diabetes, arthritis, multiple sclerosis, osteoporosis, and muscle weakness.

MYTH: Multivitamins contain enough of everything.

WHY WE THINK THAT: "Multi" means a lot of different vitamins and minerals in adequate amounts.

THE FACTS: Most multivitamins contain enough of the basic vitamins and minerals, but they often don't have enough calcium and magnesium. If milk and dark green vegetables are not a part of

> *Most multivitamins contain enough of the basic vitamins and minerals, but they often don't have enough calcium and magnesium.*

your diet, consider taking a calcium and magnesium supplement. Most of us need 1,000 to 1,200 milligrams of calcium a day, and 350 milligrams

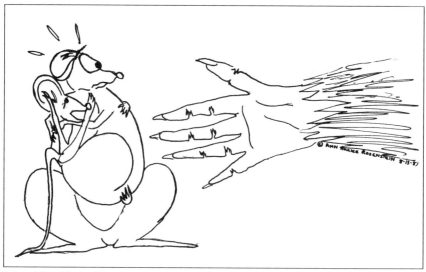

Meet Big Tom. He works over in the Supplements Division.

of magnesium. If you have enough milk and dark green vegetables in your diet, additional supplements might not be needed.

MYTH: Since I take a multivitamin, I don't need extra fish oil.
WHY WE THINK THAT: A multivitamin should do everything.

THE FACTS: While multivitamins are a good basic, unless we eat fatty fish, such as salmon, mackerel, or sardines, twice a week, we should consider taking an omega-3 fish-oil supplement. The optimum dose is 500 to 1,000 milligrams a day. Omega-3 helps prevent depression, osteoporosis, arthritis, and heart disease. If you do get enough omega-3 from your diet, you might be able to skip taking a fish oil supplement.

MYTH: The best vitamins and supplements cost a lot.
WHY WE THINK THAT: We often get what we pay for.

THE FACTS: We don't need fancy vitamins that come with extra *We don't need fancy vitamins.* ingredients or time-release additives. Stick with well-known brands, and consult a physician to be sure you are getting exactly what you need.

What to take away

- The best source of vitamins and minerals are whole, natural foods.
- Since we don't always have the best diet, we might need supplements.
- A multivitamin is a good basic and is generally enough when combined with a good diet.

29. SUPER FOODS

Cauliflower is nothing but cabbage with a college education.

— Mark Twain

Many of us believe there are foods that are just ordinary foods and then there are foods that are "super foods." In reality, most food consumed in its pure form is a good food. Yet there are some foods that offer a lot of nutrition in small packages.

Imagine super foods, powerful enough to help us lower our cholesterol, reduce our risk of heart disease and cancer, and even lift our spirits, all without side effects. We would stock up on a lifetime supply. Well, there are life-altering real super foods available in our local supermarket: whole, unrefined, unprocessed foods rich in the macronutrients, vitamins, and minerals that our bodies need.

"The effect that diet can have on how you feel today and in the future is astounding," says nutritionist Elizabeth Somer, author of *Nutrition for a Healthy Pregnancy, Food & Mood,* and *The Essential Guide to Vitamins and Minerals.*

There are life-altering real super foods available in our local supermarket.

"Even people who are healthy can make a few tweaks and the impact will be amazing," Somer says. "I'd say that 50%-70% of suffering could be eliminated by what people eat and how they move: heart disease, diabetes, cancer, hypertension can all be impacted."

We don't need specific foods for specific ailments. A healthy diet that incorporates a variety of super foods will help us maintain our weight, fight disease, and live longer. One thing the super foods all have in common is that they are real, unprocessed food. Fortified potato chips are not found in the super-food category!

Some "super foods" are:

- Beans
- Blueberries

- Broccoli
- Oats

- Oranges
- Pumpkin

260

- Salmon
- Soy
- Spinach

Spices:
- Curry
- Cardamom
- Cinnamon
- Cloves

- Tea (green or black)
- Tomatoes

- Cilantro
- Cumin
- Cayenne pepper

- Turkey
- Walnuts
- Yogurt

- Fenugreek
- Ginger
- Turmeric

Blueberries. Blueberries are a super food packed with antioxidants and phytoflavinoids. These berries are high in potassium and vitamin C, making them the top choice of

Blueberries are a super food packed with antioxidants and phytoflavinoids.

many doctors and nutritionists. Not only can they lower our risk of heart disease and cancer, they are also anti-inflammatory. When blueberries are out of season, blackberries, strawberries, raspberries, boysenberries, and grapes are good substitutes. All berries are packed with antioxidants and phytoflavinoids, but the king of berries is the blueberry.

"Inflammation is a key driver of all chronic diseases, so blueberries have a host of benefits," says Ann Kulze, MD, of Charleston, SC, author of *Dr. Ann's 10-Step Diet: A Simple Plan for Permanent Weight Loss and Lifelong Vitality.* When selecting berries, note that the darker they are, the more anti-oxidants they have. "I tell everyone to have a serving (about one-half cup) every day," Dr. Kulze says. "Frozen are just as good as fresh. Include lots of other fruits and vegetables in the diet as well and remember that the more color the fruits and vegetables have, the more antioxidants and phytoflavinoids they contain."

Fish. "We know that the omega-3s you get in fish lower heart disease risk, help arthritis, and may possibly help with memory loss and Alzheimer's," Somer says. "There is some evidence to show that it reduces depression as well."[100]

Omega-3 fats are most prevalent in fatty, cold-water fish such as wild (not farmed) salmon, herring, sardines, and mackerel. For the best results, try to have two to three servings a week. Other forms of omega-3 are available in fortified eggs, flax seed, and walnuts. These super foods

are high in monounsaturated fats, which can lower LDL ("bad") cholesterol and raise HDL ("good") cholesterol.

Soybeans. Foods made from soybeans lowers LDL cholesterol and
lower the risk of heart disease. A study reported in the *Journal of the
American Medical Association*[101] showed that a diet of soy fiber, protein
from oats and barley, almonds, and spreads from plant sterols lowered
cholesterol as much as statins, the most widely prescribed cholesterol
medicine. Tofu, soymilk, or edamame (fresh soybeans) are better than
soy powder. Soy sauce won't do the trick either, since it contains a lot of
sodium. However, if there is a family history of breast cancer, eating
extra soy is not recommended.

Fiber. Foods high in fiber keep
our weight down, our LDL cholesterol low, and reduce the risk for
cancer, diabetes, and heart disease.
A diet high in fiber will help maintain healthy cholesterol and blood

> *Foods high in fiber keep our weight down, our LDL cholesterol low, and reduce the risk for cancer, diabetes, and heart disease.*

sugar levels. Fiber specifically reduces the risk of colon cancer. When we
eliminate waste from our colon, fiber in our waste scrapes our intestinal
wall, so polyps don't develop. Dietary fiber makes us feel full longer, so
it's a great tool in weight management. Whole grains, beans, fruit, and
vegetables are all good sources of fiber. Add some beans to a salad.
Fresh, frozen, or dried beans are better than canned beans, which tend to
be higher in sodium.

Tea. Tea can reduce the risk of cancer and keeps cholesterol low. The
overall antioxidant power of black tea is the same as green tea, but green
tea does contain ECGC (epigallocatechin-3-gallate), a powerful polyphe-
nol antioxidant. A recent Japanese study[102] found that men who drank
green tea regularly had lower cholesterol than those who didn't.
Researchers in Spain and the United Kingdom have also shown that
ECGC can inhibit the growth of cancer cells. For a double health benefit,
replace sugary sodas with tea in the diet.

Calcium. Calcium builds strong bones and prevents osteoporosis.
Calcium is found in dairy products or supplements. Some studies show
that calcium helps with weight loss. Here are the daily amounts of
calcium recommended by the USDA:

- Age 9 to 18: 1,300 mg
- Age 19 to 50: 1,000 mg
- Age 51 and over: 1,200 mg

Chocolate. Finally, the best super food of all; dark chocolate!! Yes! New research has shown that dark chocolate is packed with

The best super food of all; dark chocolate!

antioxidants and can lower blood pressure. Look for chocolate with 60% or higher cocoa content; the darker, the better. In addition, the darker it is, the lower the fat and sugar content. Now that's my kind of health food!

Foods, however, are not a substitute for pharmaceutical medicines. Eating a balanced diet of non-processed foods will give us the nutrition, minerals, and vitamins that we all need, and will offset the risks of acquiring many chronic conditions, but there are no foods that will cure or reverse a disease once we have it. If you have cancer, heart disease, or diabetes, it is important to continue with a good wholesome diet and to also consult medical professionals about other therapies.

MYTH: If I eat blueberries or other unprocessed, unrefined foods, I will not get cancer, diabetes, or heart disease.

WHY WE THINK THAT: The media puts out sound bites about foods and what they can do for us all the time. We want to believe we can make ourselves immune to frightening diseases by eating certain things.

THE FACTS: Foods can be like cigarettes. There are people who have never smoked and yet they still get lung cancer; it just doesn't happen very often, only in 10-15% of all lung cancer cases.[103] In the United States, 90% of lung cancers in men and 80% of lung cancers in women are attributed to smoking.[104] Similarly, people who eat junk food and avoid fresh fruits and vegetables run a higher risk of acquiring heart disease, cancer, diabetes, and obesity and at a much earlier age. Poor eating habits and poor food choices cause premature aging and loss of the ability to remain active and independent.

We all have a 100% chance of dying. It is how well we live until then that we can control. If we eat a whole-food diet and exercise, our chances of living a longer, more independent life increase. Good diet

> We all have a 100% chance of dying. It is how well we live until then that we can control.

and exercise will lower the risk of acquiring chronic diseases. If we are lucky enough to live to a ripe old age, we will enjoy our time so much more if we are healthy and independent.

I saw the impact of exercise and healthy eating habits, or the lack of them, had on two members of my family. My grandmother and my great-aunt were about the same age. My grandmother loved sweet, sugary foods and starches, and didn't like physical activity. Her sister-in-law, my great-aunt, ate whole foods and enjoyed physical activity. My grandmother and my aunt died in the same year. My grandmother was just a few weeks shy of her 100th birthday and my aunt was 98 years old.

Here is the difference: my grandmother died in a nursing home where she had lived for more than 20 years, while my aunt died in her home where she had lived since 1949, with a full tank of gas in the car, as she had plans to take a trip. My grandmother ate the equivalent of bland baby food and slept 22 hours a day and my aunt ate normal foods and was lucid most of the day. My grandma had no teeth and my aunt had all of hers. My grandmother had been dependent on others for decades while my aunt was dependent on others for only a few months.

What to take away

- Foods high in antioxidants will help improve health.
- Super foods are not a replacement for pharmaceuticals.
- Super foods can reduce our risks for chronic diseases but will not make us immune to them.

30. MEAL PLANNING

The remarkable thing about my mother is that for thirty years she served us nothing but leftovers. The original meal has never been found.

— Calvin Trillin

You don't have to cook fancy or complicated masterpieces — just good food from fresh ingredients.

— Julia Child

Meal planning is an organized way to decide in advance what you and your family will eat over a period of time, generally one to two weeks. It is best to eat between three and six meals a day. If the time between meals is longer than four to five hours, plan to add a healthy snack on those days. Pre-planning our meals can help us eat more nutritiously, reduce our trips to the grocery store, and save time and money once we are at the store.

Menu Planning Tips

- We can use our cookbooks to plan several main meals, or we can find easy nutritious recipes online and then enter them on a menu planner. Plan some quick meals for busy nights. Double some recipes that freeze well and save half for other busy nights when there isn't time to cook. Also, plan for the possibilities of leftovers and include a "leftovers" night in the plan.

  Pre-planning our meals can help.

- Check the pantry for all the ingredients called for in the chosen recipes. Write down all the ingredients not in the pantry that are needed to complete the recipes. If you are running low on certain basic items, add these to the grocery list as well.

- List the basics used to make breakfasts, lunches, and snacks, such as eggs, cereal, bread, tuna, milk, and yogurt. List plenty of fruits and vegetables. These become our staples.
- Post the list on the refrigerator and add to it as the supply of foods runs low or as other things are needed.
- Take the list to the store and stick to it. We save money by not making impulse buys. However, don't be so rigid that you pass up a good sale item or an item you wish to try. Sticking to a list also helps to stop impulsive buying when shopping on an empty stomach.

> *Don't be so rigid that you pass up a good sale item or an item you wish to try.*

- Post the menu planner in the kitchen. Refrigerator magnets work well for this. Write down page numbers from recipe books for quick reference. This way, whoever gets home first can get dinner started. The first few times you do this, it will seem awkward and time-consuming. But that is how new behaviors feel until we become faster at the planning process. The rewards are worth it. Save the menus and grocery lists and use them again in a few weeks.

You can make the following examples into word processing documents to be printed for easy reference whenever a meal-planning form or shopping list is needed. You can customize the form to meet your family's needs.

	Breakfast	Lunch	Dinner	Snack
Monday				
Tuesday				
Wednesday				
Thursday				
Friday				
Saturday				
Sunday				

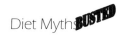

Shopping List
Produce
Bakery/bread
Baking goods
Oils, shortening
Seasonings
Pasta, grains, dried beans
Ethnic
Canned foods
Condiments
Deli

Shopping List
Frozen
Cereals/snacks
Paper/plastic
Milk, cheese, yogurt, dairy
Pets
Beverages
Laundry, cleaning
Other

What to take away:

- Meal planning isn't difficult and it pays dividends.

CONCLUSION

I get enough exercise just pushing my luck and jumping to conclusions.

— Unknown

Myths about nutrition will always come and go, but now that we know what makes a healthy food, what the macronutrients are, and how they are used by our bodies, we will be able to make intelligent choices.

Some huckster will always be out there trying to sell us the next "magic pill." Most such miracles come in the form of juices, pills, or powders. However, we now know that juices contain simple carbohydrates which, to our bodies, are just more sugar. While a juice may contain vitamins and nutrients, it will still elevate our insulin. If you are a person who already has high sugar levels, this would be counterproductive. Pills and powders only make us dependent on that product and do nothing to help educate us to change our lifestyle.

We now know that our bodies need a balance of all of the macronutrients in their most wholesome forms. So, when we are served a plate full of salad, endless servings

> *Our bodies need a balance of all of the macronutrients in their most wholesome forms.*

of bread sticks, and endless bowls of pasta, we realize we are overloading on carbohydrates and missing essential proteins and fats.

Now, when someone tells us, "Don't eat dairy products because they will make you fat," we know better. We know that dairy foods are a good source of protein, vitamin D, calcium, good fats, and essential carbohydrates. We know that too many calories make us fat.

We now know that foods fuel our bodies, and that when we consume processed and refined food or eat artificial forms of the real thing, we are depriving our bodies of valuable resources, just like fueling a precision-made car with inferior gasoline. By consuming foods that are altered from their wholesome state, we give our bodies inferior materials that place a burden on our immune systems and make us vulnerable to preventable, chronic ailments.

No matter what the experts say or sell, if we consume more calories than we use, we will become overweight. It doesn't matter if the calories are from superior or inferior sources or if they are carbohydrates, proteins, or fats; excess calories will *always* be stored as fat.

If we want to be healthy, we need to eat foods that are as wholesome and natural as they can be, and eat them in balanced amounts. All we really need to do is recognize that if the advertisement sounds too good to be true, it is. Just eat right and exercise!

> *If we want to be healthy, we need to eat foods that are as wholesome and natural.*

This is my contribution and effort to help offset the obesity crises. If after reading this book, you the reader still have questions and concerns, please visit my website at www.dietfitnessdiva.com.

Sigh. Got to go buy some food. A mouse hung itself in my fridge and left a note, "Can't live like this."

— Ustas

NOTES

1. Kaiser Health News. 2010. http://www.statehealthfacts.org/ comparebar.jsp?ind=90&cat=2
2. Americans Missing the Boat on Fitness. 2004. Nutrition Health Review http://www.thefreelibrary.com/Americans+missing+the+boat+on+fitness.-a0135663805
3. TLC. 2007. Inside Bookhaven Obesity Clinic — Rescue Me. Original air date 4-22-2007
4. TLC. 2007. Big Medicine Obesity Surgery: 5-28-2007.
5. Hawkes, N. 2008. Obesity fuels "boy-boob" problem. Timesonline. http://www.timesonline.co.uk/tol/life_and_style/men/article3964936.ece
6. 75 Percent of Obese People say they eat healthy. 2006. Associated Press MSNBC http://www.msnbc.msn.com/id/14140990/
7. Fox News. 2004, Atkins Dieters Booted by Restaurant for Eating Too Much Meat. http://www.foxnews.com/story/0,2933,118207,00.html
8. Weinstein, Amy R. et al. 2008. The Joint Effects of Physical Activity and Body Mass Index on Coronary Heart Disease Risk in Women. Arch Intern Med 168(8), 884-890.
9. Weinstein, Amy R. et al. 2008. The Joint Effects of Physical Activity and Body Mass Index on Coronary Heart Disease Risk in Women. Arch Intern Med 168(8), 884-890.
10. Taylor, J. 2005. Whether you're fat or thin; fitness is key factor, (May 21, 2005) Yakima Herald Republic.
11. Stapleton Peta & Sheldon, Teri. 2010. A Randomized Clinical Trial of a Meridian-Based Intervention for Food Cravings with Twelve Month Follow-up http://www.eftuniverse.com/index.php?option=com_content &view=article&id=3575&Itemid=2071. (8-10-2010).
12. Spiller, G. 2001. CRC Handbook of Dietary Fiber in Human Nutrition. CRC Press, Boca Raton FL.
13. Lierre, K. 2009. The Vegetarian Myth, Food, Justice and Sustainability. Flashpoint Press, Crescent City CA
14. Shai, I. 2008. Weight Loss with a Low Carbohydrate, Mediterranean, or Low Fat Diet. New England Journal of Medicine. 359:229-241
15. Esumi H, Ohgaki H, Kohzen E, Takayama S, Sugimura T. 1989. Induction of lymphoma in CDF1 mice by the food mutagen, 2-amino-1-methyl-6-phenylimidazo[4,5-b] pyridine. Japanese Journal of Cancer Research; 80(12):1176-1178.
16. Adamson RH, Thorgeirsson UP. 1995. Carcinogens in foods: Heterocyclic amines and cancer and heart disease. Advances in Experimental Medicine and Biology; 369:211-220.
17. Smith, J. 2008. Effects of marinades on the formation of heterocyclic amines in grilled beef steaks. Journal of Food Science, 73(6):T100-T105.
18. Keys, A. 1970. Coronary Heart Disease in Seven Countries. American Heart Association, New York, NY.
19. Study Fails to Link Saturated Fat, Heart Disease. 2010. American Journal of Clinical Nutrition. 92: 458-459
20. Calbom, C. 2005. The Coconut Diet: The secret ingredient that helps you lose weight while you eat your favorite foods. Warner Books. New York, NY.
21. Valtin, H. 2002. Drink at least eight glasses of water a day. Really? Am J Physiol Regul Integr Comp Physiol 283: R993–R1004.
22. Negoianu, D. & Goldfarb, S. 2008. Just add water. The Journal of the American Society of Nephrology. 19:.1041-43.
23. Negoianu, D. & Goldfarb, S. 2008. Just add water. The Journal of the American Society of Nephrology. 19:.1041-43.
24. Wojtek J Chodzko-Zajko, David N Proctor, Maria A Fiatarone Singh, et al. 2009. Nutrition and Athletic Performance, Medicine & Science in Sports & Exercise: Volume 41(3):709-731.
25. Diet Water? Get Real. 2009. http://hab913.com/bottled-water-brands/diet-water-get-real/ (8-10-2010).
26. Heller, S. 2010. Get Smart. Johns Hopkins University Press Baltimore, MD.

27. Beverage Digest. 2008. Beverage Digest Fact Book 2008: Statistical Yearbook of Non-Alcoholic Beverages. Bedford Hills, NY.

28. Wyshak G. 2000. Teenaged Girls, Carbonated Beverage Consumption, and Bone Fractures. Arch Pediatr Adolesc Med. 154:610-613.

29. Antonio, J. 2005. Juvalution: Fitness and Weight Loss through Functional Coffee. Basic Health Publications. Laguna Beach, CA.

30. Mayo Clinic. 2010. Caffeine Information. http://www.mayoclinic.com/health/caffeine/an01211

31. Walter Willett, 1994. Coffee and Coronary Heart Disease. A New Problem with Old Brew? [Editorial] Annals of Epidemiology 4(6):497-498

32. Grobbee, D., Rimm, E., Giovannucci, E., Colditz, G., Stampfer, M., Willett, W. 1990. Coffee, caffeine and cardiovascular disease in men. The New England Journal of Medicine 323:15, 1026-1032.

33. Salvaggio, A. et al. 1991. Coffee and Cholesterol, an Italian Study, American J Epidemiology 134(2):149-156.

34. World Health Organization. 2010. Lexicon of alcohol and drug terms.

35. Caffeine does not Influence calcium absorption 2001. http://www.obgyn.net/NewsRx/general_health-Bone_Health-20010924-5.asp

36. Lloyd, T., Rollings, N., Kieselhorst, K., Eggli, D., Mauger, E. 1998. Dietary Caffeine Intake is not correlated with adolescent bone gain. Journal of the American College of Nutrition, 17(5): 454-457.

37. Arab, L. 2010. Epidemiologic Evidence on Coffee and Cancer. Nutrition & Cancer, 62(3), 271-283.

38. American Cancer Society Medical and Scientific Committee. 1996. Guidelines on diet, nutrition and cancer. Cancer J. for Clinicians, 41(6):334-8.

39. AFIC 2010. MYTHS and FACTS about Caffeine http://www.afic.org/MYTHS%20and%20FACTS%20about%20Caffeine.htm Barista Guru. 2010. Coffee Myths. http://www.baristaguru.com/coffeemyths.html

40. Denby, N. 2007. Fluid, Why you need it and how to get enough. British Dietetic Association http://www.bda.uk.com/foodfacts/fluid.pdf

41. Goldbohm RA, Hertog MG, Brants HA, van Poppel G, van den Brandt PA. 1996. Consumption of black tea and cancer risk: A prospective cohort study. JNCI; 88(2):93–100.

42. Female Drinkers Less Likely to Gain Weight. 2010. Tufts University Health & Nutrition Letter, 28(3), 3-4.

43. Armstrong, E. 2005. The Cholesterol Scam. http://www.treelight.com/health/healing/Cholesterol.html

44. Armstrong, E. 2005. The Cholesterol Scam. http://www.treelight.com/health/healing/Cholesterol.html

45. Fernandez M.L. 2006. Dietary cholesterol provided by eggs and plasma lipoproteins in healthy populations. Curr Opin Clin Nutr Metab Care 9:8-12.

46. Kritchevsky, D. 1958. Cholesterol. Wiley, New York, NY.

47. University of Warwick. 2006. Sleep Deprivation Doubles Risk of Obesity in Both Children and Adults. Science Daily. Retrieved.

48. Sears, B. 1995. The Zone: A dietary road map. Reagan Books, New York.

49. Brehm,B. & D'Alessio, D. 2008 Benefits of High-Protein Weight Loss Diets, Enough Evidence for Practice? Current Opinion in Endocrinology, Diabetes and Obesity 115(5), 416-421.

50. Sok-Ja, J. Manson, J., Sesso, H., Buring, J., Simin, L. 2003. A Prospective Study of Sugar Intake and Risk of Type 2 Diabetes in Women. Diabetes Care 26, 1008-1015.

51. Zakim, D., & Herman, R. 1968. Fructose metabolism II. American Journal of Clinical Nutrition, 21: 315-319.

52. Elliot, S., Keim, N., Stern, J., Teff, K., & Havel, P. 2002. Fructose, Weightgain and the Insulin Resistance Syndrome. American Journal of Clinical Nutrition. 76(5):911-922.

53. Sears, W. 2006. Sugar. http://www.askdrsears.com/html/4/T045000.asp#T045007. Retrieved 23 Sep 10.

54. Canninton, H. 2003. Sugar: The Sweetest Poison. New Dawn.
http://www.sweetlife.com.au/Sugar_The_Sweetest_Poison.pdf
55. Men's Health Magazine. 2010. The 20 Worst Foods in America.
http://eatthis.menshealth.com/slide/8-worst-drink?slideshow=185560#title. retrieved 12-14-10.
56. Calvin, L. 2007. Spinach. http://www.ers.usda.gov/AmberWaves/June07/Features/Spinach.htm
57. Environmental Protection Agency. 2004. What you need to know about mercury in fish and
shellfish? http://www.epa.gov/waterscience/fish/files/MethylmercuryBrochure.pdf.
58. Environmental Protection Agency. 1997. Mercury Study Report to Congress.
http://www.epa.gov/ttncaaa1/t3/reports/volume6.pdf.
59. Heller, S. 2010. *Samantha Heller's Nutrition Prescription for boosting brain power and
optimizing total body health.* John Hopkins University Press. Baltimore, MD.
60. Chambers, C. 2010. Happy Halloween http://www.bellaonline.com/articles/art13943.asp
61. Cooperman, T. 2010. Nutrition Bars (Energy Bars, Fiber Bars, Protein Bars, Meal Replacement
Bars, Snack Bars and Whole Food Bars. Consumerlab.com
62. Study finds inaccurate labels on health bars. 2001 *New York Times* News Service.
http://www.intelihealth.com/IH/ihtIH/WSIIIW000/333/7228/338174.html
63. Caamano,N. 2009. Energy Bars, the good, the bad and the ugly. *Pointe 10*(5):46-8.
64. Applegate, L. 2002. *Encyclopedia of Sports and Fitness Nutrition.* Prima Lifestyles; Roseville,
CA.
65. Bauer, B. 2009. What is Kombucha tea? What are the health benefits of Kombucha tea?
http://www.mayoclinic.com/health/kombucha-tea/AN0165
66. Solomon, N. 2004. *Noni Juice, how much, how often, for what?* Direct Source Publishing; Orem,
UT.
67. Warner, J. 2004. Eat your way to a spicier sex life.
http://www.webmd.com/webmddiet/news_articles/spicier_sex_life.html.
68. Hirsch, A. 200*What flavor is your personality: Discover who you are by looking at what you eat.*
Sourcebooks; Naperville, IL.
69. Torres, E. 2000. The Taste of a Woman.
http://www.salon.com/sex/feature/2000/09/18/taste_woman/index1.html
70. Saltzman EA, Guay AT, Jacobson J. 2004. Improvement in erectile function in men with organic
erectile dysfunction by correction of elevated cholesterol levels: a clinical observation. *J Urol 172*:
255-258.
71. Ludwig, D. and Currie, J. 2010. The Association between Pregnancy Weight Gain &
Birthweight: A within Family Comparison. *The Lancet, Early Online Publication, 5 August 2010.,
doi:10.1016/S0140-6736*(10)60751-9.
72. Facts for Families 2008. Obesity in children and teens. American Academy of child and
adolescent psychiatry; facts for families no. 79
http://www.aacap.org/galleries/FactsForFamilies/79_obesity_in_children_and_teens.pdf
73. Bergman, D. 2005. Experts seek to debunk baby food myths.
http://www.msnbc.msn.com/id/9646449/ns/health-kids_and_parenting/.
74. Brandeis, R. 2006. Strategies for dealing with picky eaters.
http://www.connectwithkids.com/tipsheet/2006/277_apr19/pediatric/060419_picky.shtml#ref
75. Butte, N., 2006. *Development of an international growth standard for preadolescent and
adolescent children.* International Nutrition Foundation for United Nations University Press;
Tokyo, Japan.
76. Ludwig, D. 2007. *Ending the Food Fight; Guide your child to a healthy weight in a fast
food/fake food world.* Houghton Mifflin; Boston MA
77. Butte, N., 2006. *Development of an international growth standard for preadolescent and
adolescent children.* International Nutrition Foundation for United Nations University Press;
Tokyo, Japan.
78. University of Southampton 2007, (September 10). Food Additives Linked To Hyperactivity In
Children, Study Shows. *Science Daily*. Retrieved
79. Tucker, J., 2009. Detox Diets are Rubbish say BDA http://www.ukmedix.com/weight-
loss/detox_diets_are_rubbish_say_bda4347.cfm

80. Mitchell, B. 2006. Scientist warn detox fads a "waste of money" *Irish Examiner* http://archives.tcm.ie/irishexaminer/2006/01/04/story886935423.asp

81. The Dubious Practice of Detox. 2008. *Harvard Women's Health Watch.* 15(9): 1-3

82. BBC News. 2006. What's the point of detoxing? *BBC News magazine.* http://news.bbc.co.uk/2/hi/uk_news/magazine/4574912.stm

83. Sine, R. 2009. Detox Diets; Purging the Myths. http://www.webmd.com/diet/features/detox-diets-purging-myths

84. Dangour, A., Lock,K., Hayter,A., Aikenhead, A., Allen,E., and Uauy,R. 2010. Nutrition-related health effects of organic foods: a systematic review. *Am. J. Clinical Nutrition 92*: 203-210.

85. Leifert, C. (2007). Eat your words, all who scoff at organic food. www.timesonline.co.uk/tol/new/uk/health/article 2753446.ece

86. Hakkinen, S., & Torronen, A. 2000. Content of flavonols and selected phenolic acids in strawberries and Vaccinium species: Influence of cultivar, cultivation site and technique. *Food Research International, 33*:6, 517-524.)

87. Feridon, M. 2006. Organic Food: Buying more safety or just peace of mind? A critical review of the literature. *Critical Reviews in Food Science and Nutrition, 46*(1), 23-56.

88. Organic Trade Association. 2010. Industry Statistics and Projected Growth. http://www.ota.com/organic/mt/business.html. Retrieved 23 Sep 10.

89. Ho, MW. 2007. Scientists Find Organic Agriculture Can Feed the World & More. Institute of Science in Society. http://www.i-sis.org.uk/organicagriculturefeedtheworld.php. Retrieved 22 Sep 10.

90. Goldstein, M. 2002. *Controversies in food and nutrition.* Greenwood Press Westport, CT.

91. Public Law 101-624, Title XVI, Subtitle A, Section 1683.

92. Carlisle, J. 2000. National Survey: U.S.D.A. Organic Food Labels are Misleading. http://www.nationalcenter.org/PROrganicFood500.html]

93. Fillion, L., Arazi, S. 2002. Does organic food taste better? A claim substantiation approach. *Journal of Nutrition and Food Science. 32*(4), 153-157.

94. Dangour AD, Dodhia SK, Hayter A, Allen E, Lock K, Uauy R. 2009. Nutritional quality of organic foods: a systematic review. *Am J Clin Nutr. 90.*

95. Woese K et al. 1997. A comparison of organically and conventionally grown foods -results of a review of the relevant literature. *J Science Food and Agric 74*(3): 281-293.

96. *Am J Clin Nutr* (July 29, 2009). doi:10.3945/ajcn.2009.28041]

97. Miller, J. 2004. Organic frenzy. The Corner on National Review Online. http://www.consumerfreedom.com/news_detail.cfm/h/2334-busting-the-myth-of-organic-food.

98. Wexler, S. 2008. 6 Myths about organic food. *Marie Claire. 3*

99. Starkey, J. 2008. American Dietetic Association Welcomes The Coca-Cola Company as an ADA Partner. http://www.thebeverageinstitute.com/includes/The%20Coca-Cola%20announcement%203-1-08~%20Final.pdf

100. Somer, E. 1999. *Food & Mood: The Complete Guide to Eating Well and Feeling Your Best, Second Edition.* Holt Paperbacks, New York.

101. Jenkins, D., Kendall, C., Marchie, A., et al. 2003. Effects of dietary Portfolio of Cholesterol-lowering Foods Vs. Lovastatin on Serum Lipids and C-Reactive Protein. *JAMA 290*(4): 502-510.

102. Kuriyama, S., Shimazu, T., Ohmori, K., Kikuchi, N., Nakaya, N., Nishino, Y., Tsubono, Y., Tsuji, I., 2006 Green Tea Consumption and Mortality Due to Cardiovascular Disease, Cancer and all Causes in Japan: The Ohsaki Study. *JAMA 296*(10): 1255-1265.

103. Scagliotti, G. et al. 2009. Nonsmall cell lung cancer in never smokers. *Current Opinion in Oncology. 21*(2):99-104.

104. Alberg AJ, Samet JM. 2003. Epidemiology of lung cancer *Chest, 123*(1 Suppl):21S–49S Brownson RC, Alavanja MCR, Caporaso N, Berger E, Change JC. 1997. Family history of cancer and risk of lung cancer in lifetime non-smokers and long-term ex-smokers. *International Journal of Epidemiology; 26*(2):256–263.

GLOSSARY

abdominal fat fat that is distributed between the thorax (rib cage) and pelvis.

adipocytes fat cells.

atherosclerosis the buildup of plaques containing cholesterol and lipids on the innermost layer of the walls of large- and medium-sized arteries.

blood glucose glucose in the blood stream; blood sugar.

body mass index (BMI) the standard measure of body fat. BMI is based on an individual's weight relative to their height, and calculated by multiplying the individual's weight in pounds by 703 and then dividing that number by the individual's height in inches, squared. The units of BMI are kilograms per meter squared.

cardiovascular disease (CVD) a disease of the heart and blood vessels; any abnormal condition characterized by dysfunction of the heart and blood vessels.

childhood (pediatric) obesity though the term *childhood obesity* is commonly used, the U.S. Centers for Disease Control and Prevention (CDC) refrain from using the term "obesity" in relation to children and adolescents. Instead, the condition is referred to as *overweight.*

childhood overweight a child is classified as *overweight* if their weight ranks above the 95th percentile for their age. This represents the most severe weight classification for children and corresponds to a BMI of at least 30, the same indicator used to classify adult obesity. A term used by the U.S. Centers for Disease Control and Prevention to describe childhood (pediatric) obesity.

cholesterol soft, waxy substance manufactured by the body and used in the production of hormones, bile acid, and vitamin D. It is present in all parts of the body, including the nervous system, muscle, skin, liver, intestines, and heart. Cholesterol regulates membrane fluidity, functions as a precursor molecule in various metabolic pathways, and, as a constituent of low-density lipoproteins (LDL), may contribute to arteriosclerosis.

277

congestive heart failure condition marked by weakness, edema (fluid retention), and shortness of breath that is caused by the inability of the heart to maintain adequate blood circulation in the peripheral tissues and the lungs.

Cushing's syndrome syndrome caused by an increased production of hormone from a tumor of the adrenal cortex or of the pituitary gland. Cushing's syndrome is characterized by obesity and weakening of the muscles.

diabetes usually refers to *diabetes mellitus,* a metabolic disorder marked by increased blood glucose and often accompanied by excessive discharge of urine and persistent thirst. Discussion of other, non-nutritional kinds of diabetes is outside the scope of this book.

diabetes mellitus disease causing significant elevation of blood sugar due to deficient insulin production or action.

dyslipidemia condition marked by abnormal concentrations of lipids or lipoproteins in the blood, including lipid levels that are either higher or lower than normal, which is often a result of obesity.

endocrinology study of the glands and hormones of the body and their related disorders.

ephedrine sympathomimetic drug that, among its other effects, stimulates the generation of body heat (thermogenesis) and increases the heart rate, both of which have been thought to be signs of increased metabolism, thus ephedrine has been used in so-called diet pills.

extreme obesity defined by a BMI greater than or equal to 40.

fatty liver disease inflammation of the liver due to excessive fat deposits.

hirsutism abnormal, excessive growth of a male pattern of hair in women.

hyperinsulinemia presence of excess insulin in the blood.

hypertension abnormally elevated blood pressure; high blood pressure.

hyperthyroidism overactive thyroid.

hypoglycemia abnormally low level of glucose in the blood.

hypothyroidism underactive thyroid.

infertility absent or diminished fertility; the persistent inability to conceive a child.

insulin polypeptide hormone secreted by the islets of Langerhans in the pancreas. Insulin regulates the metabolism of carbohydrates and fats, especially the conversion of glucose to glycogen, which lowers the blood glucose level. Insulin can be synthetically created for use in the medical treatment and management of diabetes mellitus.

LAP band (laparoscopic adjustable gastric banding) surgical option to treat obesity that involves placing an inflatable band around the upper stomach, creating a small gastric pouch that limits food consumption and creates a feeling of fullness. The band can be adjusted over time to meet individual patient needs.

lipids organic (carbon-containing) substances that do not dissolve in water. Lipids, together with proteins and carbohydrates, constitute the principal structural components of living cells. Body lipids include fats, waxes, phospholipids, cerebrosides, and related/derived compounds.

lipoproteins molecules made of protein and fat that have many purposes in the body. Many enzymes and cell structure components, as well as HDL and LDL, are composed of lipoproteins.

low-carbohydrate (low-carb) common designation of food containing less than average carbohydrates. The FDA is aware that many processed food manufacturers are making reduced-carb claims in response to consumer interest in popular low-carbohydrate diets, but FDA guidelines for regulating such claims have not yet been established.

low-density lipoprotein (LDL) lipoprotein found in blood plasma that is composed of a moderate proportion of protein, a little triglyceride, and a high proportion of cholesterol. High LDL increases the risk of developing atherosclerosis. Also referred to as "bad" cholesterol.

malnutrition poor nutrition due to an insufficient or poorly balanced diet. Malnutrition can also refer to faulty digestion or utilization of foods.

metabolic syndrome disorder characterized by a cluster of health problems including obesity, high blood pressure, abnormal lipid levels, and high blood sugar.

metabolism chemical processes occurring within a living cell or organism that are necessary for the maintenance of life. During

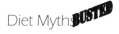

metabolism, some substances are broken down to yield energy for vital processes while other essential substances are synthesized.

normal weight ideal weight range for a given height. A BMI between 18.5 and 24.9 Kg/M^2 is the normal weight range for all people.

obesity excessive amount of body fat in relation to lean body mass; a body weight that is 30% over ideal weight for a specified height; BMI of 30 or greater

osteoarthritis form of arthritis, occurring mainly in older persons, that is characterized by chronic degeneration of the cartilage of the joints. Also called degenerative joint disease.

ovary female reproductive organ that produces eggs, estrogen, and progesterone.

overweight body weight higher than the ideal weight range but not obese. The overweight range for BMI is between 25 and 29.9. May be due to increased body fat and/or increased lean muscle.

peptides any of various natural or synthetic compounds containing two or more amino acids linked by the carboxyl group of one amino acid to the amino group of another.

pharmacotherapy treatment of disease through the use of drugs.

pituitary gland that lies at the base of the brain and controls growth, the ovaries and testes, the thyroid, the adrenal glands, and milk production.

polycystic ovary syndrome (PCOS) most common hormonal syndrome in reproductive-age women, often associated with obesity. PCOS, an accumulation of incompletely developed follicles in the ovaries, is characterized by irregular menstrual cycles, multiple ovarian cysts, and hirsutism, and often results in infertility.

prevalence total number of cases of a disease in a given population at a specific time.

reduced-carbohydrate (reduced-carb) common designation for food containing less than average carbohydrates. The FDA is aware that many processed food manufacturers are making reduced-carb claims in response to consumer interest in popular low carbohydrate diets, but FDA guidelines for regulating such claims have not yet been established.

sedentary having low activity/exercise levels.

sibutramine prescription drug used for the management of obesity that can help reduce food intake. It may be used for weight loss and maintenance of weight loss, in conjunction with a reduced-calorie diet.

sleep apnea disease that often affects overweight and obese people or those having an obstruction in the large airways, an abnormally small throat opening, or a neurological disorder. Sleep apnea causes repeated, temporary stoppage of breathing during sleep.

stroke sudden loss of brain function caused by disruption of the blood supply to the brain, by either a blockage or rupture of a blood vessel. Also called *cardiovascular accident* (CVA).

thyroid gland in the neck that produces hormones designed to regulate the body's metabolism and organ function.

triglycerides type of fat found in blood and some foods. Triglycerides are the most common type of fat in the body, are a major source of energy, and commonly circulate in the blood in the form of lipoproteins.

type II diabetes most common form of diabetes mellitus. Type II diabetes occurs when the body is resistant to the action of insulin and the pancreas cannot make sufficient insulin to overcome this resistance. Type II diabetes is often associated with obesity.

underweight weighing less than the ideal weight range; less than normal, healthy, or required weight; BMI less than 18.5.

waist circumference measurement of distance around the waist, which may be used as an obesity evaluation tool to assess abdominal fat.

BIBLIOGRAPHY

Agatston, A. 2003. *The South Beach Diet: The Delicious, Doctor-Designed, Foolproof Plan for Fast and Healthy Weight Loss.* Rodale. Emmaus, Penn.

Alexander, C. 1998. *The Endurance: Shackleton's legendary Antarctic expedition.* Caroline Alexander; in association with the American Museum of Natural History. Knopf. New York, NY.

Armstrong, L.E. 2002. Caffeine, body fluid-electrolyte balance, and exercise performance. *International Journal of Sport Nutrition and Exercise Metabolism, 12*(2):189-206.

Atkins, R, 2003. *Atkins for Life: The Complete controlled Carb Program for Permanent Weight Loss and Good Health.* St. Martin Press; New York. NY.

Atkins, R. 1972. *Dr. Atkins' Diet Revolution.* Bantam. New York, NY.

Babey, S. H., Jones, M., Yu, H., & Goldstein, H. 2009. Bubbling over: Soda consumption and its link to obesity in California. UCLA Health Policy Research Brief PB2009-5, 1-8.

Barter P, Gotto AM, LaRosa JC, Maroni J, Szarek M, Grundy SM, Kastelein JJ, Bittner V, Fruchart JC; 2007. Treating to New Targets Investigators. HDL cholesterol, very low levels of LDL cholesterol, and cardiovascular events. *N Engl J Med. 357*(13):1301-10.

Bellisari, A. 2008. Evolutionary origins of obesity. *Obesity Review, 9*(2), 165-180.

Blair, S.N. & Nichaman, M.Z. 2002. The public health problem of increasing prevalence rates of obesity and what should be done about it. *Mayo Clinic Proceedings, 77*(2), 109-113.

British Broadcasting Company. 2006. What's the point of detoxing? *BBC News Magazine.* 3 Jan. 2006. http://news.bbc.co. uk/go/pr/fr/-/1/hi/magazine/4574912.stm. 27 Nov. 2009.

Cheeseman, M. 2008. Stormy SEAS ahead for cholesterol-lowering combo. *Inpharma Weekly, 1648,* 13.

Chen L, Appel LJ, Loria C, Lin PH, Champagne CM, Elmer PJ, Ard JD, Mitchell D, Batch BC, Svetkey LP, Caballero B., et al. 2009. Reduction in consumption of sugar-sweetened beverages is associated with weight loss: the PREMIER trial. *American Journal of Clinical Nutrition 89*:1-8.

Christian, B., McConnaughey, K., Bethea, E., Brantley, S., Coffey, A., Hammond, L., Harrell, S., Metcalf, K., Muehlenbein, D., Spruill, W., Brinson, L., & McConnaughey, M. 2004 *Pharmacology Biochemistry and Behavior, 78*(1), 121-127.

Consumers Union. 2008. Sweeteners: How the brands measure up. *Consumer Reports 72(*10), 16-17.

Deardorf, J. 2010 Rise Eat and Shine What you eat for breakfast can make or break your day. Here's the right way to get started. *Minneapolis Star Tribune Lifestyle, Health and Wellness.* http://www.startribune.com/lifestyle/health/95805469.html ?elr=KArks7PYDiaK7DUvDE7aL_V_BD77:DiiUiD3aPc:_Yyc:aULPQL7PQLanchO7DiUr

Diamond, H. 1985. *Fit For Life.* Warner Books. New York. NY.

Dietary Reference Intakes for Energy, Carbohydrates, Fiber, Fat, Fatty Acids, Cholesterol, Protein, and Amino Acids (Macronutrients). 2005. National Academics Press. Washington D.C.

Doliver, M. 2005. People tell one story about weight, while the scale tells quite another. *Adweek, 46*(47), 25.

Edelbaum, M. 2008. Is soda bad for bones? Three reasons to think before you drink. *Eating Well Magazine.* 28 May 2008. http://shine.yahoo.com/channel/food/is-soda-bad-for-bones-3-reasons-to-think-before-you-drink-176623. 27 Nov. 2009.

Facchini, F., Fiori, G., Toselli, S., Pettener, D., Battistini, N., & Bedogni, G. 2003. Is elbow breadth a measure of frame size in non-Caucasian Populations? A study in low- and high-altitude Central-Asia Populations. *International Journal of Food Sciences & Nutrition, 54*(1), 21-26.

Fat acceptance. 2008. *Weightloss Health & Beauty Online.* 20 Aug. 2008. http://onlinehealthandbeauty.blogspot.com/2008/08/fat-acceptance.html 27 Nov. 2009.

Fiore, E. 1965. *The L-C Diet.* The Ridge Press. New York, NY.

Flora, C. The protein-hunger connection. *Psychology Today* 23 Jan. 2006. http://www.psychology today.com/node/20417. 27 Nov. 2009.

Frederick, C. 1965. *Dr. Carlton Frederick's Low-Carbohydrate Diet.* Award Books. New York NY.

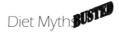

Frisancho, A. R. & Flegel, P. N. 1983. Elbow breadth as a measure of frame size for US males and females. *The American Journal of Clinical Nutrition, 37*(2), 311-314.

Fulgoni V, 3rd. 2008. High-fructose corn syrup: everything you wanted to know, but were afraid to ask. *American Journal of Clinical Nutrition 88*:1715S

Gregg. G. www.youngfatandfabulous.com

Guignon, A. N. 2008. What are we drinking? *RDH: The National Magazine for Dental Hygiene Professionals, 28*(1), 32-36.

Hansson GK. 2005. Inflammation, Atherosclerosis, and Coronary Artery Disease *N Engl J Med 352*:1685.

Harding, K. 2009. *Lessons From The Fat-O-Sphere: Quit Dieting and Declare a Truce With Your Body.* Perigee Book; New York, NY.

Harding, K. www.therotund.com

Harper Collins *Webster Dictionary.* 2003. Harper Torch New York, NY.

Harris, W. 2008. You are what you eat applies to fish, too. *Journal of the American Dietetic Association, 108*(7), 1131-1133.

Hochman, A. 2008. Top six myths about bottled water. *Marie Claire.* http://www.marieclaire.com/life/healthy/health-tips/bottled-water-myth. 27 Nov. 2009.

Janket, S. J., Manson, J. E., Sesso, H., Buring, J. E., & Liu, S. 2003. A prospective study of sugar intake and risk of type 2 diabetes in women. *Diabetes Care, 26*(4), 1008-1015.

Jekyll and Hyde Grasshoppers Teach Us about Obesity http://eureka.australianmuseum.net.au/9DICC4-957718A-7A38583EE03EC6C2?DISPLAYENTRY=true

Jones, K. E., Johnson, R. K., & Harvey-Berino, J. R. 2008. Is losing sleep making us obese? *Nutrition Bulletin, 33*(4), 272-278.

Kipple, Kenneth F. 1997. *Plague, Pox and Pestilence: Disease in History.* Weidenfeld and Nicholson: London.

Kulze, A. 2008. *Dr. Ann's 10-step Diet: A Simple Plan for Permanent Weight Loss and Lifelong Vitality.* Top Ten Wellness and Fitness, New York.

LaBerge, A. F. 2008. How the ideology of low fat conquered America. *Journal of History of Medicine and Allied Sciences, 63*(2), 139-177.

Li, D. 2010. New Jersey woman attempting to become world's fattest lady. *New York Post.* www.nypost.com

Lindqvist, A., Baelemans, A., & Erlanson-Albertsson, C. 2008. Effects of sucrose, glucose and fructose on peripheral and central appetite signals. *Regulatory Peptides, 150*(1-3), 26-32.

Linn, R. 1977. *The Last Chance Diet...When Everything Else Fails.* Lyle Stuart, New York, NY.

Lupu, A. 2006 The hunger hormone: Is it really that easy to control obesity or anorexia? *Softpedia.* 17 Jul. 2006. http://news.softpedia.com/news/The-Hunger-Hormone-Is-it-Really-that-Easy-to-Control-Obesity-or-Anorexia-30006.shtml. 27 Nov. 2009.

McGraw, P. 2003. *The Ultimate Weight Solution: The 7 keys to Weight Loss freedom.* Free Press, New York NY.

Mozaffarian, D., Rimm, E., & Herrington, D. 2004. Dietary fats, carbohydrate, and progression of coronary atherosclerosis in postmenopausal women. *American Journal of Clinical Nutrition, 80*(5) 1175-1184.

National Institute of Health. 2007. *Fact Sheet: Alcohol Dependence (Alcoholism).* http://www.nih.gov/about/researchresultsforthepublic/AlcoholDependence Alcoholism.pdf. 27 Nov 2009

Neuharth, D. 2004. *Secrets you keep from yourself: How to stop sabotaging your happiness.* St. Martin's Press. New York, NY.

Ornish, D. 1990. *Dr. Dean Ornish's Program For Reversing Heart Disease: The only System Scientifically Proven to Reverse Heart Disease without Drugs or Surgery.* Random House. New York, NY.

Palca, J. 2007. Scientists identify a gene linked to obesity. *National Public Radio.* 12 Apr. 2007. http://www.npr.org/templates/story/story.php?storyId=9545915. 27 Nov. 2009.

Pollan, M. 2008. *In defense of food: An eater's manifesto.* Penguin Press. New York, NY.

Schlosser, E. & Wilson, C. 2006 *Chew on this: Everything you don't know about fast food.* Houghton Mifflin, Boston, MA.

Shai, I., Schwarzfuchs, D., Henkin, Y., Shahar, D. R., Witkow, S., Greenberg, I., Golan, R., Fraser, D., Bolotin, A., Vardi, H., Tangi-Rozental, O., Zuk-Ramot, R., Sarusi, B., Brickner, D., Schwartz, Z., Sheiner, E., Marko, R., Katorza, E., Thiery, J., Fiedler, G. M., Blüher, M., Stumvoll, M., & Stampfer, M. J. Weight loss with a low-carbohydrate, Mediterranean, or low-fat diet. *New England Journal of Medicine, 359*(3), 229-241.

Shell, E. 2002 *The hungry gene: The science of fat and the future of thin.* Atlantic Monthly Press. New York, NY.

Simon, M. 2006. *Appetite for Profit: How the food industry undermines our health and how to fight back.* Nation Books, New York, NY.

Sine, R. 2006. Detox diets: purging the myths. *WebMD.* 12 May 2009. http://www.webmd.com/diet/features/detox-diets-purging-myths. 27 Nov. 2009.

Somer, E. 1995. *Nutrition for a healthy pregnancy: the complete guide to eating before, during, and after your pregnancy.* H. Holt and Co. New York, NY.

Somer,E. 1992. *The Essential Guide to Vitamins and Minerals.* Harper Perennial; New York, NY.

Somer,E. 1995. *Food and Mood: The complete guide to eating well and feeling your best.* Holt, New York, NY.

Super Juices Review and Compare. 2004. *Journal of Agricultural and Food Chemistry, 52,* 4026-4037.

Spiers, E. 2008. Devil's food. *Fast Company.* 28 Jan. 2008. http://www.fast company.com/magazine/122/devils-food.html. 27 Nov. 2009.

Stevens, J., Cai, J., Evenson, K. R., & Thomas, R. 2002. Fitness and fatness as predictors of mortality from all causes and from cardiovascular disease in men and women in the lipid research clinics study. *American Journal of Epidemiology, 156*(9), 832-841.

Swithers, S. E., & Davidson, T. L. 2008. A role for sweet taste: calorie predictive relations in energy regulation by rats. *Behavioral Neuroscience, 122*(1), 161-173.

Valtin, H. 2002. "Drink at least eight glasses of water a day" Really? Is there scientific evidence for "8 x 8"? *American Journal of Physiology Regulatory, Integrative, and Comparative Physiology, 283,* 993-1004.

Wang, Y., Beydoun, M. A., Liang, L., Caballero, B., & Kumanyika, S. K. Will all Americans become overweight or obese? Estimating the progression and cost of the US obesity epidemic. *Obesity, 16*(10), 2323-30.

Wansink, B. 2006. *Mindless Eating: Why we eat more than we think.* Bantam Books, New York, NY.

Weaver, K. L., Ivester, P., Chilton, J. A., Wilson, M. D., Pandey, P., & Chilton, F. H. 2008. The content of favorable and unfavorable polyunsaturated fatty acids found in commonly eaten fish. *Journal of the American Dietetic Association, 108*(7), 1178-1185.

Willoughby, M. Big corpses pose unusual challenges for morgues. *Orlando Sentinel.* 4 Jan. 2008.

Yang, Z. & Hall, A. G. 2008. The financial burden of overweight and obesity among elderly Americans: The dynamics of weight, longevity, and health care cost. *Health Services Research, 43*(3), 849-868.

Zelman, K. 2010. Not all Carbs are Created Equal http://www.webmd.com/diet/features/not-all-carbs-are-created-equally

Zinczenko, D. & Goulding, M. 2007. *Eat this, not that! Thousands of simple food swaps that can save you 10, 20, 30 pounds or more!* Rodale, Emmaus, Penn.

Zinczenko, D. & Gouling, M. 2008. *Eat this, not that! For kids! Be the leanest, fittest family on the block!* Rodale, Emmaus, Penn.

INDEX

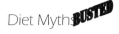

ABOUT THE AUTHOR

Ann Rosenstein is a certified fitness instructor and personal trainer with certifications from ACE, AFAA, AEA, Schwinn Cycle and a Pilates certification from the Physicalmind Institute. Ann has been teaching group fitness, water aerobics, and weight training since 1989. She also has a BA and MA from the University of Minnesota and works as a reference librarian for the Dakota County Library System in Minnesota. Besides *Diet Myths Busted*, Ann has written *Water Exercises for Parkinson's*, *Water Exercises for Fibromyalgia*, *Water Exercises for Osteoarthritis*, and *Water Exercises for Rheumatoid Arthritis*.

Ann practices what she preaches in this book with her husband Leo and children, Sarah and Ben. Favorite family activities are working out, outdoor biking, cross-country skiing, and rollerblading. Ann will address your questions or concerns about nutrition or fitness interactively through her website: www.dietfitnessdiva.com.

Please visit and ask away!